"Written by the pre-eminent leaders in the field of schizophrenia research with decades of clinical experience, this user-friendly book offers a cutting-edge, evidence-based compendium of all things psychosis – symptoms, treatment, diagnosis, and prognosis. Written for both the avid clinician and concerned family member, the authors seek to instill hope and discuss the effectiveness of treatment to change the course of this potentially devastating disease and, when possible, prevent the onset of illness altogether. A must-have for all psychiatrists!"

–Anna Yusim, MD, chief psychiatrist, Upper East Side Psychiatry; lecturer, Yale University Department of Psychiatry; distinguished fellow, American Psychiatric Association; author, fulfilled

"The title of this wonderful book, 'Understanding and Caring for People with Schizophrenia: Fifteen Clinical Cases', does not begin to do justice to the breadth of topics and issues it covers. Besides focusing on the symptomatic presentation and treatment options (including medication, psychotherapy, and psychoeducation) for the prodromal, first-episode, and chronic stages of Schizophrenia, it expertly covers a wide range of other important topics, such as the heritability of Schizophrenia, violence and suicide, the impact of drug use, as well as sections focusing on important symptoms such as the various types of delusions (including exotic ones such as the Capgras delusion), hallucinations, negative symptoms and cognitive deficits. What makes the information contained in this book come alive is its reliance on interesting and compelling case material to illustrate the various topics, which should make this book especially appealing to students, clinicians-in-training, and patients and family members."

–Michael First, MD, professor of Clinical Psychiatry, Columbia University

"Dr. Girgis and colleagues have produced a very useful addition to the literature on schizophrenia. The case history format makes the disease and its associated problems, come alive. The book will be especially useful for trainees in all mental health disciplines who wish to better understand this fascinating, if sometimes devastating, disease. The book is also accessible for individuals with schizophrenia and their families who wish to do a deeper dive into its details and to see that some cases are indeed treatable. Strongly recommended."

–E. Fuller Torrey, MD, author, *Surviving Schizophrenia and American Psychosis*

"These internationally renowned mental health experts have written a remarkable book – one that is compelling to read, compassionate, and highly educational. Written without jargon, the text is easily understood by the general public while at the same time providing concise clinical pearls that will help experienced clinicians provide even better care of their patients. The approach of starting each chapter with a detailed case illustration – often in the patient's voice – followed by discussion is both absorbing and illuminating. Each case provides a resounding message of hope – that recent advances in mental health have done much to enhance the prognosis and lives of those with schizophrenia."

–Brian A. Fallon, MD, MPH, professor of Clinical Psychiatry; director of the Center for Neuroinflammatory Disorders; and Biobehavioral Medicine and director of the Lyme and Tick-Borne Diseases Research Center, Columbia University

"Written by leading researchers of schizophrenic spectrum disorders, using 15 case studies, Drs. Girgis, Brucato and Lieberman provide wisdom and illuminate the complexity and heterogeneity of schizophrenia. The rich and eloquently written case vignettes capture the human dimension of the illness while at the same time deepening one's clinical understanding, and provide evidence as to the effectiveness of treatment at different phases of the illness. This scholarly book is a must read for clinicians, academicians, and anyone interested in schizophrenia."

–Ali Khadivi, PhD, ABAP, professor of Psychiatry and Behavioral Sciences, Albert Einstein College of Medicine

UNDERSTANDING AND CARING FOR PEOPLE WITH SCHIZOPHRENIA

This book challenges professional and public misconceptions of schizophrenia as an illness with intractable symptoms and inexorable mental deterioration, educating clinicians and researchers on the effectiveness of treatment to change the course of or prevent the onset of illness.

The authors illustrate such effectiveness through fifteen case studies examining psychosis in diverse clients. These case studies are divided into the three phases of the illness – onset, chronic and recurrent, and treatment (refractory and residual) with accompanying analyses of the causes, symptoms, interventions, and treatments. By depicting patients at different clinical stages of the illness, with accompanying explanations of how they got to that point, what might have been done to avoid – or has been done to achieve – this outcome, the reader will gain an appreciation of the nature of the illness and for the therapeutic potential of currently available treatments.

Readers will learn about the various clinical aspects of schizophrenia and treatment including diagnosis, prognosis, clinical presentation, suicide risk, cognitive deficits, stigma, medication management, and psychosocial interventions.

Ragy R. Girgis, MD, MS, is an associate professor of Clinical Psychiatry at the Columbia University Department of Psychiatry and New York State Psychiatric Institute. He has published 80 peer-reviewed scientific papers and has also recently authored *On Satan, Demons, and Psychiatry: Exploring Mental Illness in the Bible*, published in 2020.

Gary Brucato, PhD, is an associate research scientist in the Department of Psychiatry at Columbia University Irving Medical Center in New York City. An expert on psychosis and violence, he has published nearly 40 peer-reviewed journal articles on these topics. This is his second book. He was also the author, with Dr. Michael H. Stone, of *The New Evil: Understanding the Emergence of Modern Violent Crime*, published in 2019.

Jeffrey A. Lieberman, MD, is the Lawrence C. Kolb Professor and Chairman of Psychiatry, Columbia University, Vagelos College of Physicians and Surgeons, and the director of the New York State Psychiatric Institute. He has published hundreds of peer reviewed journal articles, including some of the most seminal articles in the field of schizophrenia. In addition, Dr. Lieberman has written or edited 11 books on mental illness, psychopharmacology, and psychiatry.

UNDERSTANDING AND CARING FOR PEOPLE WITH SCHIZOPHRENIA

Fifteen Clinical Cases

*Ragy R. Girgis, Gary Brucato,
and Jeffrey A. Lieberman*

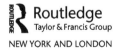

Routledge
Taylor & Francis Group

NEW YORK AND LONDON

First published 2021
by Routledge
52 Vanderbilt Avenue, New York, NY 10017

and by Routledge
2 Park Square, Milton Park, Abingdon, Oxon OX14 4RN

Routledge is an imprint of the Taylor & Francis Group, an informa business

© 2021 Taylor & Francis

The right of Ragy R. Girgis, Gary Brucato, and Jeffrey A. Lieberman to be identified
as authors of this work has been asserted by them in accordance with sections 77 and 78
of the Copyright, Designs and Patents Act 1988.

Library of Congress Cataloging-in-Publication Data
Names: Girgis, Ragy R., author. | Brucato, Gary, 1978– author. |
Lieberman, Jeffrey A., 1948– author.
Title: Understanding and caring for people with schizophrenia:
fifteen clinical cases / Ragy R. Girgis, Gary Brucato, Jeffrey A. Lieberman.
Description: New York, NY: Routledge, 2021. |
Includes bibliographical references and index. |
Identifiers: LCCN 2020019541 (print) | LCCN 2020019542 (ebook) |
ISBN 9780367370107 (hardback) | ISBN 9780367369996 (paperback) |
ISBN 9780367854652 (ebook)
Subjects: MESH: Schizophrenia | Case Reports
Classification: LCC RC514 (print) | LCC RC514 (ebook) |
NLM WM 203 | DDC 616.89/8–dc23
LC record available at https://lccn.loc.gov/2020019541
LC ebook record available at https://lccn.loc.gov/2020019542

ISBN: 978-0-367-37010-7 (hbk)
ISBN: 978-0-367-36999-6 (pbk)
ISBN: 978-0-367-85465-2 (ebk)

Typeset in Bembo
by Newgen Publishing UK

CONTENTS

INTRODUCTION

The professional and public view of schizophrenia is one of intractable symptoms and inexorable mental deterioration born from images of the homeless, media depictions of psychotic killers, and the entertainment industry's exploitation of mental illness for dramatic purposes. However, research over the last three decades has provided evidence of the effectiveness of treatment to change the course and even prevent the onset of the illness. To illustrate this underappreciated reality, this book will provide 15 different stories/essays of psychosis divided into the three phases of the illness, namely onset, chronic and recurrent, and treatment-refractory and residual. Each essay will describe case histories of some of our patients, each dealing with aspects of psychosis specific to that phase of the illness. These cases will be based on the decades of experiences of the authors. While providing a narrative on each case, the authors will editorialize about aspects of psychosis described above.

The goal of this book will be to disabuse clinicians of the therapeutic nihilism that has historically pervaded the field by educating health professionals and the interested lay public about psychosis and many of the important clinical aspects of psychosis, such as diagnosis (i.e., positive symptoms, negative symptoms, etc.), self-injury and suicidality, cognitive deficits, stigma, the importance of medications, duration of untreated psychosis, dangerousness, the prodrome, treatment refractoriness and clozapine, social downward drift, and psychosocial interventions, through real-life clinical cases. By depicting patients at different clinical stages of the illness, with accompanying explanations of how they came to that point, what might have been done to avoid – or has been done to achieve – this outcome, the reader will gain an appreciation of the nature of the illness and for the therapeutic potential of currently available treatments.

Our objective is for this book to be a resource for an academic and professional audience. We find that many mental health practitioners and students in health-related fields including psychiatry, psychology, social work, and many other fields of medicine interested in learning more about, or required to learn about, psychosis are grossly under- or miseducated about psychosis. Our primary goal is to provide an engaging yet educational account of what psychosis is really like, as well as to educate them about the important clinical aspects of psychosis, such as treatment, symptoms, prognosis, diagnosis, etc. A secondary target audience would be patients and their family members and friends who may not fully understand what it means to have schizophrenia and would like to learn more about it. Further, although treatment refractoriness is a substantial problem in psychosis, we aim to instill hope and realistic expectations in clinicians, patients and their family members/friends who may have much less experience with psychosis and, in our experience, tend toward a much more discouraged and nihilistic view of psychotic disorders.

Importantly, while the patients and situations described in this book are informed by our combined extensive experience seeing patients, all patient descriptions are anonymized in order to protect their confidentiality. Some cases may reflect composites of patients who may illustrate generic characteristics of the illness and its clinical care.

Finally, to introduce ourselves, Ragy R. Girgis, MD, MS, is an Associate Professor of Clinical Psychiatry at the Columbia University Department of Psychiatry and New York State Psychiatric Institute. He is an expert in severe mental illness, and in particular schizophrenia, with a focus on brain imaging as well as the development of experimental treatments. He has published 80 peer-reviewed scientific papers and has also recently authored *On Satan, Demons, and Psychiatry: Exploring Mental Illness in the Bible*, published by Wipf and Stock in 2020.

Gary Brucato, PhD., is an Associate Research Scientist in the Department of Psychiatry at Columbia University Irving Medical Center in New York City. An expert on psychosis and violence, he has published nearly 40 peer-reviewed journal articles on these topics. He was also the author, with Dr. Michael H. Stone, of *The New Evil: Understanding the Emergence of Modern Violent Crime*, published by Prometheus Books in 2019.

Dr. Jeffrey A. Lieberman is the Lawrence C. Kolb Professor and Chairman of Psychiatry, Columbia University, Vagelos College of Physicians and Surgeons, and the Director of the New York State Psychiatric Institute. He has published hundreds of peer reviewed journal articles, including some of the most seminal articles in the field of schizophrenia. In addition, Dr. Lieberman has written or edited 11 books on mental illness, psychopharmacology, and psychiatry, including *Shrinks: The Untold Story of Psychiatry* (Little Brown, 2015), as well as the textbook *Psychiatry*, currently in its 4th edition, published by John L. Wiley, and *The American Psychiatric Publishing Textbook of Schizophrenia*.

PART I

Onset (Early Identification and Prevention)

1

USING PSYCHOTHERAPY AND MEDICATIONS TO TREAT A TEENAGER WITH PRODROMAL SYMPTOMS

"Fran" was a 17-year-old conservative Mormon female who was referred to our clinical high-risk for psychosis (CHR) clinic by her private psychiatrist in the context of possible attenuated positive symptoms. She and her family trace their roots back to the first Mormon communities in Western New York. Her ancestors migrated from New York to Ohio to Missouri and then to Utah where they settled in an exclusively Mormon community. Fran's family lived in Utah for many generations. Fran was born in Utah. She was born at term and without complications. She achieved her developmental milestones on time and was a generally healthy child. Fran enjoyed a life immersed in a conservative Mormon culture and community. She had many friends and a robust social life, along with her family and many other families in her community.

At the age of ten, Fran's father, who was a Mormon clergyman, was asked to lead a Mormon community in another state. Although unhappy and some-what frightened about the move since neither had ever lived anywhere except for in Utah and in an exclusively Mormon community, Fran and her mother, a homemaker, were obedient to the requests of the church. Therefore, Fran and her parents left their community in Utah and moved to a small community in another state.

The move was difficult for Fran. She was exposed to different cultures and lifestyles, substantially different from her own. The move was made more difficult by her mother's very adverse reaction to the move. Away from her family and friends, all of whom were still in Utah, Fran's mother became very sad and anx-ious. She felt out of place and was unable to deal with her feelings of isolation. Her depression, anxiety, and feelings of isolation were worsened by the lack of avail-ability of Fran's father, who was extremely busy, working 7am–10pm seven days a week, building and tending to his young congregation. The difficulties that Fran's mother faced prevented her from being available, both emotionally and practically, to Fran during the difficult transition period.

By the age of 15, Fran began to experience substantial depression and anxiety. Her depression and anxiety began to affect her performance at school. Therefore, Fran began to see a therapist, and then eventually a psychiatrist. She participated in weekly psychotherapy, as well as monthly medication management. Fran saw her therapist and psychiatrist for approximately two years before she was referred to our clinic. The reason for the referral was that Fran's therapist and psychiatrist were not sure why their treatments were not having a substantial effect, and they suspected, though were not sure, that "something else may be going on."

When we first met Fran we were struck by how shy she was, as well as by how intelligent she was. She appeared young for her age. She rarely made eye contact. Her speech was very sophisticated, clear, and eloquent, although she had minimal spontaneous speech. She described her mood as "depressed" and had a blunted affect. She stated that, in the previous two years, people had given her feedback that she looked tired and apathetic, sometimes asking, "Are you okay?" Fran reported anxiety since age ten, characterized by nervousness when having to socialize or be in public places, with some school refusal. She reported a serious period of depression in the tenth grade, characterized by not leaving her room, crying, decreased appetite and subsequent weight loss, low self-esteem, low energy, impaired concentration, and intermittent suicidal ideation, with images of hanging herself or overdosing, with two attempts to drown herself to death, without success, prompting hospitalization. While her mood had improved substantially since this episode, she continued to experience chronic dysphoria and low motivation.

Fran described herself as anxious in social situation, but capable of maintaining a few good friends at a time despite this. In the year before presenting to our clinic, in the context of growing suspiciousness and low self-esteem, she began avoiding all social interactions, making excuses to avoid engagements with friends. She spent most of her time alone or with family, dancing in her room, reading, watching movies with her father, working on her homework, viewing television, and sleeping.

Despite her difficulties, Fran was in talented and gifted classes in elementary school and in honors classes in middle school. She was also a very successful and high achieving student from kindergarten through the ninth grade, earning straight "A"s. Upon entering her current school, her grades declined to mostly "B"s, which she and her family attributed to diminished interest and motivation. She also cited a period of hospitalization for suicidality and difficulty catching up with her work post-discharge. She had never failed a subject. Fran's goal was to pursue further education in Japanese dance, with hopes of someday dancing for an eminent dance company and touring the country.

Fran described positive relationships with both of her parents, although she described some guilt about having been irritable with them at times across her lifetime. She also generally felt that they were not paying enough attention to her because she was a failure and was letting them down as a result of her dream to pursue Japanese dance, as well as because of her psychiatric condition. Her perception was that her parents would not approve of her wanting to pursue Japanese dance as a profession, but would have preferred her to pursue a career in academia. In addition, although her family was educated and knowledgeable about mental illness, she was self-conscious about it given the stigma surrounding mental illness.

The clinic to which Fran was referred was for individuals at clinical high-risk for psychosis. Schizophrenia usually develops in the mid- to late-teens or early twenties (1). It often begins with a period of attenuated symptoms (2). This period before schizophrenia fully develops is referred to as a "prodrome." During this period, people experience delusions and hallucinations like people with full psychosis, though they are attenuated in nature, meaning that people who have them can still be convinced that their delusions or hallucinations are not real, i.e., they have less than 100% conviction. For example, prodromal individuals may have persecutory thoughts, such as that they are being watched, or the FBI is out to get them. However, they will maintain at least some insight, so that they can be convinced, for example, that the FBI is not out to get them, or that they may not be watched. Prodromal individuals may also have abnormal perceptual experiences like hallucinations, but understand that they are actually coming from their mind and are not real phenomena. For example, a prodromal person may hear a muffled voice, but understand that it is coming from their own mind.

Similarly, many prodromal individuals experience negative symptoms and cognitive deficits. These deficits are similar in quality to individuals with syndromal schizophrenia, though of a lesser intensity (2). For example, prodromal individuals may experience anhedonia, anergia, amotivation, alogia, apathy, and avolition. However, all of these would generally be experienced with less intensity than how someone with syndromal schizophrenia would experience them. Similarly, individuals with prodromal psychosis may experience cognitive impairments such as impaired attention, short-term memory, or executive functioning. These cognitive deficits tend to be milder than those experienced by individuals with schizophrenia.

Prodromal individuals also often experience a decline in academic and social functioning (2). However, this impairment in functioning is generally not as severe as that experienced by individuals with schizophrenia and may not be apparent until very close to when they actually develop syndromal schizophrenia. Furthermore, prodromal individuals very often experience other nonspecific symptoms such as depression and anxiety. Many of these people will have already received psychiatric care for comorbid conditions, such as major depressive disorder, obsessive compulsive disorder, or other anxiety disorders, before their diagnosis of prodromal psychosis. This period can last between days and years, though very uncommonly lasts more than two to two-and-a-half years (2, 3).

The prodrome is, however, a retrospective diagnosis as it can only be made once it is certain that someone has schizophrenia or psychosis, since not everyone with attenuated delusions and hallucinations develops schizophrenia. In fact, upwards of almost 8%–20% of the population has attenuated or full psychotic symptoms at some point in their lifetime (4, 5). Many of these people simply have schizotypal personality disorder or other conditions. Therefore, when someone is prospectively, or in real time, identified as having attenuated delusions and hallucinations, they are considered to be at "clinical high-risk" for psychosis, or CHR. Approximately 30% of CHR individuals actually develop a full, syndromal schizophrenia (2, 3). The word "prodromal," then, can only be given after it is known that someone has developed a psychotic disorder.

This raises three very important questions. The first is if 20% of the population has at least attenuated positive symptoms at some point in their lives, how are CHR individuals diagnosed? The second is, once someone is diagnosed as being CHR, how would one determine whether a CHR individual is more likely than another to develop a syndromal schizophrenia? Third, what becomes of the 70% of CHR individuals who do not develop a syndromal psychotic disorder?

Regarding the first question, there are two main criteria used to distinguish people who are actually at high-risk for psychosis, which is actually a very uncommon diagnosis, and people who are not. First, people are generally only considered high-risk for psychosis if their attenuated positive symptoms develop between the ages of approximately 14–30. While it is possible for someone to develop schizophrenia at another age, it is much less likely. Therefore, people are only considered high risk for psychosis if these symptoms develop between the ages of 14–30.

The second criterion has to do with time course of symptoms. As described above, many people, such as individuals with schizotypal personality disorder, have attenuated positive symptoms that began when they were very young, even as children, and basically stay stable throughout their lives. Meanwhile, we know very well that the prodromal period is a very dynamic time when symptoms develop and progress relatively quickly (i.e., within two years) to schizophrenia. Therefore, only people with attenuated positive symptoms that are new or worsening in the previous year, and between the ages of 14–30, are considered to be at high-risk for transition to a syndromal psychotic disorder (6). Further, once identified as being at high-risk for psychosis, the vast majority of individuals who will transition to a full psychotic disorder will do so within two to two-and-a-half years (~95%) (2, 3).

Regarding the second question, once someone is diagnosed as being CHR, how would one determine whether a CHR individual is more likely than another to develop a syndromal schizophrenia? Many different criteria, calculators, algorithms, and variables have been examined and developed with little consensus or true distinguishing characteristic found. However, recent research suggests that not only does the recency and intensification of positive symptoms determine who is CHR, these criteria also serve as the best prognostic indicators for the development of syndromal schizophrenia. In particular, the more positive symptoms that someone has, which are new or worsening within the previous year, the more likely someone is to develop a syndromal condition (6).

What becomes of the 70% of CHR individuals who do not develop a syndromal psychotic disorder? Many of them have persistent, attenuated positive symptoms, as observed in the so-called "Cluster A" personality disorders from the DSM-IV – namely, schizoid personality disorder, paranoid personality disorder, and, most commonly, schizotypal personality disorder (7). Attenuated positive symptoms are also occasionally observed in the so-called "Cluster B" personality disorders, especially borderline personality disorder. In a substantial minority of cases, the positive symptoms remit and the patients are left with mood and anxiety disorders (8, 9). A small minority of patients completely remit from any psychiatric condition, although this is less common.

Fran had a number of attenuated positive symptoms. She reported a longstanding sense of the world feeling unreal, with thoughts that she might actually be unconscious but alive somewhere, dreaming what appeared to be the world around her. She reported 10% conviction about this idea, at peak. In the most recent several months, these experiences prompted thoughts that she might actually have been a host for a computer, or possibly another organism, with about 10% conviction at peak. Fran reported that, across her lifetime, she had the sense that her pet fish may actually have been aliens from another planet, controlling the channels on her television, with about 30% conviction at peak. This idea had increased in the previous year to occur daily with about 50% conviction at peak. Fran reported intrusive violent images over the previous nine months of running over baby deer or shooting an arrow through a person's head, stating emphatically that she rapidly dismissed these images, which were ego-dystonic, and that she had no specific desire to act upon them. Since the eighth grade, she had the daily concern that she needed to censor her thoughts, because the pet fish in her home were transmitting her thoughts via radio waves to other planets. This concern had increased in the previous year, in terms of intensity and conviction, to 30% at peak. Fran reported daily concerns, since the tenth grade, that she might be infested with worms which cause occasional stomach upset, diarrhea, cramps, and occasional anal bleeding. This prompted anxious discussions with her parents who were uniformly able to encourage her to abandon this worry. Her conviction level had been about 25% about this idea with no increase in the previous year.

Fran did not present as guarded at any point throughout the interview process and was uniformly engaged and forthcoming. She reported concern over the previous year that other people disliked her and wished to harm her. She suggested they may have been plotting to harm her and may have been working with her pet fish. She suggested that the pet fish may have been supplying her classmates and other people in public areas with special guns that would disintegrate her hair and clothes, leaving her naked and bald, thereby exposing her to the world. She had increasing thoughts about this over the previous few months, to become daily, with about 30% conviction at peak and avoidance of some social interactions.

Fran reported several instances around age 13 of feeling that leaders of other religions were talking to her through the radio, trying to get her to change her religion, with about 50% conviction. Fran also described daily thoughts, starting about one year before presentation, with 90% conviction at peak that she would become a famous Geisha. She reported that she performed as a Geisha daily.

Fran also reported longstanding hypersensitivity to sound, especially low-pitched sounds that many other people would not hear, such as bass. Twice per week over the previous month she had heard her name called when nobody was around. One time she heard the word "ugly" and one time she heard a sound "like someone sneezing on me." Several months before her presentation she saw something in the corner of her eye which she thought was one of her pet fish flying, though she understood that would have been impossible. About two months before her presentation she began feeling a warm sensation in her stomach and hips about two times per week.

Based on her symptoms, Fran met criteria for someone at clinical high-risk for psychosis. She agreed to enroll in our clinic and began receiving weekly psychotherapy and medication management. At the time she was considering college with a goal to attend a premier dance conservatory. However, the patient's symptoms were debilitating and affecting her functioning. Fran still had her senior year of high school to complete. At the time of her presentation, it was not clear that she would have been able to graduate high school, let alone enter a prestigious college. All signs pointed toward a bad prognosis and even progression to a full psychotic illness, such as schizophrenia.

We decided to take a two-pronged approach to treating Fran. The first prong was medication management. When Fran first presented to our clinic, she was being prescribed 40mg of escitalopram, 2mg of risperidone, 10mg of olanzapine, 1500mg of divalproex sodium, and 50mg of Lamictal. She was also prescribed 0.25mg of clonazepam as needed for anxiety.

In the CHR or prodromal stages of the illness, the state of the art is to treatment comorbidities, such as anxiety and depression, as one would treat them anywhere. In addition, as patients' positive symptoms become closer to meeting full criteria for psychosis (i.e., full conviction), many physicians will often prescribe antipsychotic medications, such as olanzapine or risperidone, prophylactically. These medications can often help prevent agitation and can enhance the effect of other medications. However, paradoxically, while antipsychotic medications are very effective for syndromal schizophrenia, there remains no evidence of any intervention, including medications or otherwise, capable of preventing progression to a full, syndromal psychotic illness. One may then ask why anyone would ever prescribe antipsychotic medications to someone who is not fully psychotic, and for that matter what is the reason identifying people in the CHR/prodromal state of illness is important if there is nothing we can do in the first place.

The answer to both these questions is the same and gets at the heart of why the CHR phase is important. The first major advance in the treatment of schizophrenia occurred in the early 1950s with the discovery of antipsychotic medications (10). These medications revolutionized care for schizophrenia and lent great evidence to the notion that schizophrenia was a brain disease, rather than a result of bad parenting or weak morals. The second advance was the development and testing of clozapine in the late 1980s, as described later in this book (11).

Around the same time that clozapine became available, very important research was being conducted that suggested, and then was later confirmed, that early intervention in schizophrenia is important (12–19). Namely, that means that the earlier in their illness that someone receives antipsychotic medications the better their long-term outcome. This has now been replicated many times and is one of the most important concepts in the field of schizophrenia research. This concept is well known as "duration of untreated psychosis," or DUP for short, the goal being to minimize DUP as much as possible.

The CHR field developed in large part from the desire to minimize DUP as much as possible, because identifying people before they even develop syndromal psychosis allows one the opportunity to not only minimize DUP, which is possible, but also to potentially prevent the onset of illness. The latter is not yet possible, but a goal of the field.

However, despite the importance of starting antipsychotic medications early, there is no evidence in full psychotic or mood illnesses such as schizophrenia or bipolar disorder that a six-medication regimen, consisting of two mood stabilizers, two antipsychotic medications, one anti-anxiety agent, and one antidepressant, would be any better than one agent. Therefore, with the patient's and parents' consent, we began to slowly taper Fran's medications, starting with olanzapine. Tapering off each medication took approximately one to two months as it is generally preferable to taper off medications gradually in order to minimize withdrawal effects as well as to minimize any potential return of symptoms.

The second prong was to take a dynamic but pragmatic and personalized approach in the weekly psychotherapy. Her therapist helped her to reframe, understand, and make meaning out of her symptoms in the context of her experiences – as stories that would help her work through her challenging life circumstances. For example, her therapist helped her to reframe her thoughts that her pet fish were aliens by understanding that this could have been a story that she developed to deal with the lack of attention that she was receiving from her parents and her social isolation in general. The fish were providing the attention that she was not obtaining from her family and friend group. In addition, as a gifted and emotional dancer, Fran was very empathic and emotive. She also believed that people could read her mind. Fran's therapist helped her understand that she assumed that everyone was as empathic as her and therefore could easily read her mind, which was not true. Further, Fran's father was a prominent clergyman in the Mormon church. Fran assumed that she was embarrassing her father and felt overly judged for this. In reality, and through multiple family meetings, it became clear to Fran that her parents were extremely loving and proud of Fran and supported her decision to pursue dance as a career.

Fran and her therapist formulated a mantra for these exercises. Whenever Fran would describe a symptom such as those above, she or her therapist would say the mantra, "Be a Hiruti." The purpose of the mantra was to remind Fran of the emotional and psychological depth that she had, as exemplified by her favorite geisha Hiruti, and could use to better understand her symptoms. During one session, Fran remarked: "That person was looking at me and was mean." Her therapist replied, "Be a Hiruti." Fran was then able to develop a more nuanced understand of what may have been happening, including that the random person on the street who was looking at her with a mean expression may have been unhappy for other reasons, or sad, or thinking about something completely different than Fran.

Fran responded to her therapy and medication changes quickly and robustly. Within six months she achieved near complete resolution of her symptoms, began obtaining straight "A"s at school again, and began to engage more with friends. By the end of the year she was off nearly all her medications except for 0.5mg of risperidone and had matriculated at a premier dance conservatory. Fran and her parents were exceedingly happy with her progress and her private psychiatrist at home remarked that Fran's turnaround was one of the greatest she had ever seen.

Five years later, Fran was doing better than she had ever been. She was happily married with one child. She was teaching dance at a local theater. She was no longer taking medications and had continued in a weekly psychotherapy. While it is impossible to say for sure whether Fran's therapy and medication management had helped to avert progression to full psychosis or another condition, we were very happy for Fran and felt confident that there is hope for people suffering from symptoms thought to be harbingers of more serious psychiatric illness.

References

1.   Lieberman JA, First MB. Psychotic disorders. *N Engl J Med*. 2018;379(3):270–280.
2.   Fusar-Poli P, Borgwardt S, Bechdolf A, Addington J, Richer-Rossler A, Schultze-Lutter F, Keshavan M, Wood S, Ruhrmann S, Seidman LJ, Valmaggia L, Cannon T, Velthorst E, De Haan L, Cornblatt B, Bonoldi I, Birchwood M, McGlashan T, Carpenter W, McGorry P, Klosterkotter J, McGuire P, Yung A. The psychosis high-risk state: a comprehensive state-of-the-art review. *JAMA Psychiatry*. 2013;70(1):107–120.
3.   Brucato G, Masucci MD, Arndt LY, Ben-David S, Colibazzi T, Corcoran CM, Crumbley AH, Crump FM, Gill KE, Kimhy D, Lister A, Schobel SA, Yang LH, Lieberman JA, Girgis RR. Baseline demographics, clinical features and predictors of conversion among 200 individuals in a longitudinal prospective psychosis-risk cohort. *Psychol Med*. 2017;47(11):1923–1935.
4.   van Os J, Hanssen M, Bijl RV, Vollebergh W. Prevalence of psychotic disorder and community level of psychotic symptoms: an urban-rural comparison. *Arch Gen Psychiatry*. 2001;58(7):663–668.

5. Van Os J, Linscott RJ, Myin-Germeys I, Delespaul P, Krabbendam L. A systematic review and meta-analysis of the psychosis continuum: evidence for a psychosis proneness-persistence-impairment model of psychotic disorder. *Psychol Med.* 2009;39(2):179–195.

6. Brucato G, First MB, Dishy GA, Samuel SS, Xu Q, Wall MM, Small SA, Masucci MD, Lieberman JA, Girgis RR. Recency and intensification of positive symptoms enhance prediction of conversion to syndromal psychosis in clinical high-risk patients. *Psychol Med.* 2019:1–9.

7. Zoghbi AW, Bernanke JA, Gleichman J, Masucci MD, Corcoran CM, Califano A, Segovia J, Colibazzi T, First MB, Brucato G, Girgis RR. Schizotypal personality disorder in individuals with the Attenuated Psychosis Syndrome: frequent co-occurrence without an increased risk for conversion to threshold psychosis. *J Psychiatr Res.* 2019;114:88–92.

8. Addington J, Cornblatt BA, Cadenhead KS, Cannon TD, McGlashan TH, Perkins DO, Seidman LJ, Tsuang MT, Walker EF, Woods SW, Heinssen R. At clinical high risk for psychosis: outcome for nonconverters. *Am J Psychiatry.* 2011;168(8):800–805.

9. Schlosser DA, Jacobson S, Chen Q, Sugar CA, Niendam TA, Li G, Bearden CE, Cannon TD. Recovery from an at-risk state: clinical and functional outcomes of putatively prodromal youth who do not develop psychosis. *Schizophr Bull.* 2012;38(6):1225–1233.

10. Lehmann HE, Hanrahan GE. Chlorpromazine: new inhibiting agent for psychomotor excitement and manic states. *AMA Arch Neurol Psychiatry.* 1954;71(2):227–237.

11. Kane J, Honigfeld G, Singer J, Meltzer H. Clozapine for the treatment-resistant schizophrenic. A double-blind comparison with chlorpromazine. *Arch Gen Psychiatry.* 1988;45(9):789–796.

12. Kirch DG, Lieberman JA, Matthews SM. First-episode psychosis: Part I. Editors' introduction. *Schizophr Bull.* 1992;18(2):177–178.

13. McGlashan TH. A selective review of recent North American long-term followup studies of schizophrenia. *Schizophr Bull.* 1988;14(4):515–542.

14. Wyatt RJ. Neuroleptics and the natural course of schizophrenia. *Schizophr Bull.* 1991;17(2):325–351.

15. Perkins DO, Gu H, Boteva K, Lieberman JA. Relationship between duration of untreated psychosis and outcome in first-episode schizophrenia: a critical review and meta-analysis. *Am J Psychiatry.* 2005;162(10):1785–1804.

16. Loebel AD, Lieberman JA, Alvir JM, Mayerhoff DI, Geisler SH, Szymanski SR. Duration of psychosis and outcome in first-episode schizophrenia. *Am J Psychiatry.* 1992;149(9):1183–1188.

17. Rabiner CJ, Wegner JT, Kane JM. Outcome study of first-episode psychosis. I: relapse rates after 1 year. *Am J Psychiatry.* 1986;143(9):1155–1158.

18. Thara R, Henrietta M, Joseph A, Rajkumar S, Eaton WW. Ten-year course of schizophrenia: the Madras longitudinal study. *Acta Psychiatr Scand.* 1994;90(5):329–336.

19. Lieberman J, Jody D, Geisler S, Alvir J, Loebel A, Szymanski S, Woerner M, Borenstein M. Time course and biologic correlates of treatment response in first-episode schizophrenia. *Arch Gen Psychiatry.* 1993;50(5):369–376.

2

PERSECUTORY DELUSIONS AND THE TRANSITION FROM CLINICAL HIGH-RISK TO SYNDROMAL PSYCHOSIS

"Mr. S" had a very difficult upbringing. He was born to a single, 17-year-old mother. He was her second child. He was born at term. His father, a recent immigrant from another country, had no relationship with the mother except for the one night they spent together. Mr. S's mother had three additional children from three different men after Mr. S was born. While Mr. S was growing up his mother was rarely at home, spending most of her time at clubs and with other men at their apartments. Therefore, as an infant and toddler, Mr. S was raised primarily by his grandparents and neighbors in a public housing project. Almost everyone living in his area lived below the poverty line. Drugs were sold on nearly every street corner and murders were a weekly occurrence. Police were occasionally present but generally not involved in Mr. S's area. Life was very tough in this neighborhood. Most young people in Mr. S's area knew nothing of the outside world except what they would occasionally watch on television. Mr. S did not leave his neighborhood, until he was 16 years old, when his high school went on a field trip to Central Park. This was typical of young people growing up in Mr. S's neighborhood.

By the time that Mr. S had achieved school age his mother began spending more time at home. However, she was still generally unavailable as she had to work two jobs in order to support her five children and continued to spend most of her free time with men, many of whom she would bring to her home. Therefore, from a young age, Mr. S spent much of his time surrounded by numerous strange men.

When Mr. S was ten years old his mother befriended a man from the neighborhood whom she had met at work. He was different than most of the men with whom his mother would spend time. He had a steady job, treated Mr. S's mother with respect, and spent time with her children, including with Mr. S. In fact, Mr. S enjoyed spending time with this man. They would throw a baseball to each other outside of their building and watch baseball on television together. Every month or so the boyfriend would buy food from a popular fast food chain for Mr. S and his siblings to share.

Mr. S's mother and her boyfriend were together for several months. Over this time, Mr. S developed strong feelings for the boyfriend. He even began to call him "dad." Mr. S would look forward to seeing his mother's boyfriend and would ask his mother about when he would be visiting.

One day, about eight months after Mr. S's mother and her boyfriend began their relationship, Mr. S was walking home from school. He had been sent home early because he was developing an upper respiratory tract infection, one that he had likely contracted from his older sister who had missed school the previous three days because of her cold. As Mr. S came to his apartment door, he saw that the mother's boyfriend's bicycle (he often traveled to their home via bicycle) was leaning against the wall. Mr. S was very excited to see that the mother's boyfriend was at their apartment. When Mr. S walked into the apartment, he found his sister and his mother's boyfriend interacting in ways that appeared uncomfortable and unfamiliar to Mr. S, in a way that primarily involved touching and other types of contact in the genital and anal areas. Mr. S did not know what was happening. When his mother's boyfriend saw Mr. S, he told him that he and his older sister were simply "playing" and that they would like Mr. S to join. Mr. S did not want to join and his older sister did not look like she was having fun, but, since no other adult supervision, protection, or guidance was available, the mother's boyfriend began to involve Mr. S in their "play."

We met Mr. S when he was 19 years old. At first glance, he appeared guarded, angry, and suspicious, though otherwise appeared to be a normal looking, casually dressed teenager. He was five feet, eight inches tall, thin but athletic appearing, and had an uncanny resemblance to a famous musician. His speech was normal in rate and rhythm. He had few friends and was enrolled in a community college.

We had two initial sessions with Mr. S, each lasting two hours. Although Mr. S did at first glance appear to be relatively guarded and suspicious, he was rather charismatic and endearing. He was surprisingly open about his life and experiences, including the three years of sexual molestation that he experienced as a child and early teenager that he had never previously told anyone – his "dirty laundry" as he described it. Though open about his experiences, he was noticeably more irritable and angry when discussing this time in his life than when discussing other times in his life. Ultimately, he decided to enroll in our clinical high-risk for psychosis clinic.

On full interview, Mr. S described a number of attenuated positive symptoms. He stated that, for two years, the world felt "slowed down." He described this as if the world were "moving in slow motion, but just barely." He described this thought as intrusive and distressing and one that he would "obsess" about to the point that it would bother him. It would sometimes keep him from going outside because of how much he was thinking about it. Mr. S reported that he only believed that the world was actually "slowed down" with about 40% conviction, but also that, over the previous three months, he realized that he could revert the pace of the world to normal by clapping his hands lightly three times. He did not understand why this had an effect and sometimes thought that what he was doing was silly, but since it worked he continued to do it anyway.

Mr. S also described a number of persecutory ideas. He reported that, while he was initially happy that he looked like a famous musician, he had begun to think that this was a "curse." He explained that, because of his appearance, people were jealous of him and sometimes mistook him for this musician. He explained that large men looked at him as if they wanted to fight him to prove that they were more masculine than he is just because they thought that he was famous. Everywhere he went, Mr. S felt this scrutiny with approximately 80% conviction. He was willing to consider that his thoughts may not have been real and that people were really not looking at him or wanting to fight him. He reported that he was now socializing much less than he used to socialize, but that he was not bothered by this because he was not as interested in socializing or having friends as much as he used to be.

Mr. S described that these fears would occasionally keep him up at night. He reported feeling constantly tense, on edge, and restless. He reported that, in general, his mood was not very good and he almost always felt irritable or somewhat sad. His thoughts were often distracting to him. On occasion, Mr. S would "obsess" so much about his concerns and feel so anxious that he would feel fatigued for the remainder of the day.

Mr. S described that he would hear, since mid-adolescence, very brief, vague sounds, like voices, saying "you" or "hey you." They seemed insignificant to him; however, in the previous year, he had begun wondering, at a four to five out of ten conviction level, whether these sounds might have been people talking to him. He sensed that they came from inside of his head, so he usually dismissed these thoughts. He stated that, although the idea that these sounds may have been something other than his own mind seemed "crazy" to him, he found himself increasingly interested in the possibility. They had no significant impact on his behavior.

Mr. S also reported referential thoughts about things he would see on television about one time per month in the previous year which felt, at a conviction level of six or seven out of ten, like they were put there to "mess with" him. He described a sense over the previous year that some of the news reporters, especially on music channels, were referring to him in what they said, though not actually saying his name. He stated that no one but him would have known that they were talking to him. He reported that he entertained this idea with eight out of ten conviction.

Mr. S reported that, over the previous year, he began to have intrusive thoughts of running over people on the sidewalk with a car. He had always recognized these violent images to be products of his mind; found them distressing; wanted very intensely for them to dissipate with treatment; and had never acted on them. He emphatically stated several times during the interview that he had no intention to ever act on these; had no access to a car; could not afford a car even if he wished to acquire one; felt in control of himself; and was seeking treatment to help remain in control.

Mr. S described and exhibited some grandiose ideas, stating that he occasionally felt as if there was something special about him and that it was not a coincidence that he looked like a musician. He suggested that there was something superior and special about him, but was vague as to what it was.

Mr. S reported that he began psychiatric treatment when he was 15 years old and had been in both psychotherapy and medication management since that time. He reported that he had been given a number of different diagnoses. He reported that his first diagnosis was attention deficit hyperactivity disorder. He was given that diagnosis because of his problems with attention and distraction. He tried a number of different medications for his inattention, including amphetamines, methylphenidate, and atomoxetine. He reported that he obtained limited benefit from these medications and that his grades had been decreasing over the previous six months, though he felt that amphetamines made him feel better and gave him energy. He reported that his psychiatrist continued him on 20mg twice daily of amphetamines and he had been taking this for three years.

About two years after Mr. S was diagnosed with ADHD, he stated that he was diagnosed with depression and anxiety because of his feelings of low mood, restlessness, and anxiety/fears that people were singling him out and paying attention to him. Mr. S reported that he received diagnoses of social anxiety disorder and generalized anxiety disorder, as well as major depressive disorder because of his low and irritable mood. For these symptoms, Mr. S was prescribed a number of medications, including paroxetine, fluoxetine, gabapentin, hydroxyzine, and duloxetine. At the time of his evaluation with us, Mr. S was taking 40mg of fluoxetine as well as hydroxyzine 50mg by mouth three times a day as needed for anxiety. Mr. S reported that he did not feel that these medications were really helping him, but that his psychiatrist told him to take them.

Another diagnosis that Mr. S received shortly before presenting to our clinic was obsessive-compulsive disorder. He reported that he received this diagnosis when he told his psychiatrist and therapist about his thoughts that he felt that the world was "slowed down" and that he realized that he could return the world to its normal pace by clapping his hands lightly three times. He reported that his psychiatrist told him that his intrusive thoughts of running over people on the sidewalk with a car were also "obsessions" and therefore further evidence of his obsessive-compulsive disorder. For this, Mr. S received exposure and response prevention therapy. Mr. S reported that, while he benefited from seeing a therapist weekly, he did not feel that the exposure exercises were helpful.

The final diagnosis that Mr. S received before enrolling in our clinic was post-traumatic stress disorder. He reported that he received this diagnosis after telling his psychiatrist about his fears of people, his history of trauma, and the vague voices that he was hearing. For this, Mr. S was referred to an eye movement desensitization and reprocessing (EMDR) therapist. Mr. S reported that he tried this for one session and became so paranoid that he abruptly left before the first session had ended.

Comorbidity, or having two conditions, is very common in psychiatry, and especially in individuals at clinical high-risk for psychosis (1, 2), such as Mr. S. In general, having comorbid conditions makes one's treatment substantially more complicated. However, what makes comorbidity even more challenging in clinical high-risk patients is that not only can people have bona-fide conditions such as anxiety and depressive disorders in addition to their attenuated positive symptoms, but sometimes attenuated positive symptoms can be misinterpreted as anxiety, mood, or other disorders.

For example, Mr. S was first diagnosed with ADHD. However, people who develop psychosis, or even people with depression or anxiety, often exhibit very early signs of inattention, as did Mr. S. Unfortunately, because psychiatric diagnoses are based purely on phenomenology, and Mr. S's initial clinicians did not have the benefit of knowing whether or not he would develop another disorder, he was diagnosed with ADHD and treated with stimulant medications. Importantly, stimulant medications, such as amphetamines, are relatively contraindicated in individuals at clinical high-risk for psychosis, as they are in individuals with full psychotic disorders, and so this medication was likely not helping, and possibly hurting, Mr. S.

Anxiety disorders are also commonly diagnosed in individuals with attenuated positive symptoms. For example, Mr. S complained of "anxiety" that he was being watched and being singled out. Since Mr. S maintained some insight into his symptoms, and because he used the word anxiety, he was misdiagnosed as having social anxiety disorder when he, in fact, was experiencing attenuated persecutory delusions. These points are also relevant to his diagnosis of generalized anxiety disorder. Mr. S described feeling tense, on edge, restless and frequently worrying about people overscrutinizing or watching him. He reported irritability and some insomnia related to these feelings. As with his diagnosis of social anxiety disorder, since Mr. S maintained some insight into his symptoms, and because he used the word "anxiety," one might have misdiagnosed him with generalized anxiety disorder, when in fact his symptoms were related to the attenuated persecutory delusions that he was experiencing.

Post-traumatic stress disorder and dissociation in general are also very commonly diagnosed in clinical high-risk patients. Upwards of 10%–25% of these patients may have experienced a trauma in their lives, such as did Mr. S (3). Feelings of hypervigilance can often be used to explain attenuated persecutory delusions, and dissociation is often used to explain attenuated hallucinations. Without a context for Mr. S's symptoms, a diagnosis of PTSD would not have been unreasonable. However, given the nature of his symptoms, that most of them were not related to his trauma, and that many of them were very recent in onset, PTSD was not the most likely diagnosis for Mr. S.

Depressive disorders, especially major depressive disorder, are perhaps the most frequently diagnosed comorbid conditions in clinical high-risk patients. Many times, individuals have depressive disorders unrelated to their attenuated psychosis. In other cases, an individual's depression is, in part, precipitated by the realization of how devastating and upsetting a burgeoning psychosis can be.

Perhaps the most difficult differential diagnosis for the clinical high-risk state is obsessive-compulsive disorder. Mr. S was diagnosed with obsessive-compulsive disorder when he told his psychiatrist and therapist about his thoughts that he felt that the world was "slowed down" and that he realized that he could return the world to its normal pace by clapping his hands lightly three times. He reported that his psychiatrist told him that his intrusive thoughts of running over people on the sidewalk with a car were also "obsessions" and therefore further evidence of his obsessive-compulsive disorder. Differentiating between obsessive-compulsive disorder and clinical high-risk symptoms can be very difficult. For example, many of Mr. S's symptoms could in fact have been described as obsessions and compulsions (intrusive thoughts of running over people in his car, repeatedly thinking that the world was "slowed down" and compulsively clapping his hands lightly three times to speed up the world). Why then would one consider Mr. S's clinical picture to be more consistent with attenuated psychotic symptoms rather than obsessive compulsive disorder? There are six criteria that one could use to differentiate between obsessive compulsive disorder and attenuated positive symptoms: 1) Obsessive compulsive disorder tends to involve obsessions and compulsions that are less magical and bizarre, while obsessions and compulsions that occur in the context of attenuated positive symptoms tend to be extremely implausible, such as thinking the world is "slowed down," and that clapping could somehow make the world speed up; 2) Negative symptoms and cognitive deficits, such as the anhedonia, asociality, and inattention experienced by Mr. S, are more likely to suggest obsessions and compulsions that occur in the context of attenuated positive symptoms rather than obsessive compulsive disorder; 3) A family history of a psychotic disorder would be more likely to suggest obsessions and compulsions that occur in the context of attenuated positive symptoms rather than obsessive compulsive disorder; 4) Having other attenuated positive symptoms, such as the auditory perceptual abnormalities, attenuated grandiosity, and attenuated paranoia experienced by Mr. S would be more likely to suggest obsessions and compulsions that occur in the context of attenuated positive symptoms than obsessive compulsive disorder; 5) Symptoms that begin in the mid- to late-teens, rather than in the late childhood and early teenage years, would be more likely to suggest obsessions and compulsions that occur in the context of attenuated positive symptoms than obsessive compulsive disorder; 6) Individuals who do not respond to therapies designed for obsessive compulsive disorder, such as selective serotonin reuptake inhibitors and exposure and response prevention, would be more likely to suggest obsessions and compulsions that occur in the context of attenuated positive symptoms than obsessive compulsive disorder. While none of these criteria would necessarily individually differentiate between an attenuated positive symptom syndrome and obsessive compulsive disorder, together they could, on balance, suggest one over the other.

Based on these criteria, as well as Mr. S's complete history, Mr. S was diagnosed as being at clinical high-risk for psychosis and enrolled in our clinic. Mr. S spent approximately a year in our clinic. He became comfortable with the staff in our clinic and developed a strong alliance with his therapist. We did notice, however, that he seemed to feel more comfortable around men in our clinic and that this reflected what was happening in his personal life. He had essentially no female friends or influences at all and had even stopped interacting with his sister.

In the months after which Mr. S enrolled in our clinic, he revealed very disturbing ideas explaining his isolation from women. Namely, his experiences with being sexually molested as a child had left him distrustful and generally antagonistic toward women to the point that he had almost completely isolated himself from women altogether. Mr. S admitted to feeling the most hostile toward his sister. Mr. S explained that, although it was a man who molested him, he had begun to realize that it was his sister who was behind the molestation. Mr. S went on to say that – though he did not realize it at the time that he was being molested – he had begun to realize that his sister, like most men, was jealous that he looked like a famous musician and wanted to humiliate him. Men would want to either fight him and beat him up to show that they were superior to him, or rape him, thereby humiliating him. He described that his sister, since she was not strong enough to rape him or beat him up, would form alliances with men and harass him. Mr. S described to us that "it was all becoming clear" that the voices he was hearing were his sister and neighbors who were harassing him. He reported that whenever women would see him and realize that he looks like a famous musician they would first want to make love to him and then, when they realized that he was uninterested, ally with his sister and join in on the harassment.

Over time, Mr. S began to explain his other symptoms as occurring in the context of very systematic and interconnected delusions, rather than as isolated, unusual experiences. Mr. S revealed that his sister actually had supernatural powers and was somehow able to make the world "slow down." Her goal, as per Mr. S, was to extend his suffering and humiliation while he was being molested or humiliated, similar to how he felt that time slowed down every time his mother's boyfriend molested him when he was younger.

Over the next several months, Mr. S was treated with intense therapy and initiation of antipsychotic medications. Mr. S began to speak less and less of his desire to run over people with a car and was generally less paranoid. He re-engaged in his schoolwork and began working a part-time job. Unfortunately, during the same time period, his delusional system expanded. Mr. S explained that the vague voices that he was hearing coming from his own head began to sound more like his sister's voice and come from five to ten feet away. He reported that the voices seemed to be angrier than before and were comprised of four-letter words.

To Mr. S, the "last straw," as he described it, before he confronted his sister and moved out of their home, was when he began to realize that, not only did he look like a famous musician, but that he was famous himself. He cited the non-stop references to him on the television (this referential thinking had progressed from being limited to music channels to being on nearly all channels, even home shopping channels) and accused his sister of revealing his deepest secrets (such as about being molested) to the public.

Despite taking antipsychotic medications and working through his feelings of hostility toward women and his sister in particular, Mr. S progressed toward a full psychotic illness. Although we initiated antipsychotic medications, and they did help to some degree, there is currently no known way to prevent progression to a syndromal psychotic condition in individuals at clinical high-risk for psychosis. However, as described above, providing medications early is critical in order to decrease the duration of untreated psychosis, which, in Mr. S's case, was very short.

This case also highlights how one would determine whether a patient has become fully psychotic – i.e., whether or not they have transitioned to a syndromal psychotic disorder. While having full, 100% conviction about a positive symptom, such as a delusion, would by definition be adequate to diagnose someone with a psychotic illness, there are several other clinical observations that can suggest someone is developing or has developed a full psychotic illness. One way would be to follow the location of a patient's auditory perceptual abnormalities, if they endorse them. It is often, though not always, the case that as someone progresses from having an attenuated to syndromal auditory perceptual abnormality, the sound (whether a voice or other sound) migrates from occurring inside or very close to one's head to more definitively occurring outside of one's head, including feet or tens of feet away. This is not always the case as many individuals with schizophrenia experience voices inside of their head, but this can be a useful phenomenon to keep in mind when determining whether someone has developed a syndromal psychosis or not.

Another important sign that someone is developing a psychotic illness is the interconnectedness of their symptoms. Often, especially when people are early in the clinical-high-risk phase, their symptoms, such as paranoia, perceptual abnormalities, and other attenuated positive symptoms, are disconnected and experienced as relatively unusual, mysterious, and vague. However, as one moves toward having a full psychotic disorder, their disparate symptoms begin to coalesce around a theme and become interconnected. Mr. S, for example, initially had paranoia, grandiose ideas, and auditory perceptual abnormalities that were relatively unrelated. As he developed a full psychotic disorder, he began to make connections between the symptoms and realized how they all fit in together, forming one large narrative that made sense to him and was no longer vague. This is almost pathognomonic of the development of a psychotic disorder.

We referred Mr. S to a clinic for full psychotic illnesses closer to where he was living as he had decided to move out of his current home and neighborhood, due to his severe paranoia. Mr. S indicated to us his deep appreciation for helping him deal with his trauma and reported a desire to see us again in the future.

That time was two weeks later. Mr. S began working at the laundromat near his previous therapist's apartment, collecting and weighing the dirty laundry from the customers. The therapist was unsure what to do. We advised the therapist to choose a different laundromat if this made him or the patient feel uncomfortable.

While it is not uncommon for patients to develop attachments to their therapists and feel a strong inclination to see them after the end of a treatment, it is also not usual for patients to find their way into their therapists' personal lives, although it does happen. We never heard from or saw Mr. S again, and we never found out whether it was by happenstance or plan that Mr. S was working in the therapist's laundromat, collecting his dirty laundry.

References

1. Brucato G, Masucci MD, Arndt LY, Ben-David S, Colibazzi T, Corcoran CM, Crumbley AH, Crump FM, Gill KE, Kimhy D, Lister A, Schobel SA, Yang LH, Lieberman JA, Girgis RR. Baseline demographics, clinical features and predictors of conversion among 200 individuals in a longitudinal prospective psychosis-risk cohort. *Psychol Med*. 2017;47(11):1923–1935.
2. Addington J, Piskulic D, Liu L, Lockwood J, Cadenhead KS, Cannon TD, Cornblatt BA, McGlashan TH, Perkins DO, Seidman LJ, Tsuang MT, Walker EF, Bearden CE, Mathalon DH, Woods SW. Comorbid diagnoses for youth at clinical high risk of psychosis. *Schizophr Res*. 2017;190:90–95.
3. Grivel MM, Leong W, Masucci MD, Altschuler RA, Arndt LY, Redman SL, Yang LH, Brucato G, Girgis RR. Impact of lifetime traumatic experiences on suicidality and likelihood of conversion in a cohort of individuals at clinical high-risk for psychosis. *Schizophr Res*. 2018;195:549–553.

3

THE HERITABILITY OF SCHIZOPHRENIA AND DEALING WITH HAVING A FAMILY MEMBER WITH SCHIZOPHRENIA

"Andrea" was a 20-year-old Caucasian heterosexual female with possible attenuated psychosis who was self-referred to our clinic after learning about us online. She resided in an apartment in Manhattan, New York with her 54-year-old father, "Wilson," a former child television actor and occasional movie actor with a history of schizophrenia, and her 50-year-old mother, "Diana," who had schizoaffective disorder, as well as acromegaly, attributable to a pituitary tumor that was inoperable. Andrea's parents met at an intensive outpatient program shortly after both of them had their first psychotic episodes. Andrea's father worked in sanitation and her mother as an administrative assistant. Andrea was diagnosed with "depression" in her teens. Andrea had one sister, "Laura," who was three years younger, with whom she had a very positive relationship and who suffered from severe bulimia, overeating and vomiting at least twice a day for three years and less frequently before that. Andrea reported an extensive additional family history of mental illness including a grandfather who died in an institution in Eastern Europe for treatment-refractory psychotic mania; a maternal great aunt who killed herself via asphyxiation after the birth of her second child; a grandmother with dementia and severe alcoholism; an uncle with obsessive compulsive disorder and agoraphobia so severe that he had not left his home in 25 years; a cousin with bipolar disorder; several aunts and uncles with opioid use disorders; and a maternal great uncle with schizophrenia who had the delusion that he was able to communicate with animals. He was killed by a pack of wolves at the age of 28 when he tried to integrate himself into a pack in the wilderness outside of where he lived at the time. Andrea also had an uncle who had molested several children in his neighborhood and was serving time in prison.

Andrea reported always doing well in school, attaining a "B+" or "A−" average across her lifetime. Beginning in high school she worked during the summers, first in fast food and then in retail clothing. She was always noted to be responsible and successful in her work.

Socially, Andrea reported positive social relations prior to the time of a playground accident at age 8, which left her with a scar on the left side of her face which made her feel "ugly," greatly impacting her confidence. Afterward, she felt so ugly she should have been "locked in the bell tower" and began to grow her hair very long and keep it over the left side of her face. Shortly before presenting to our clinic, Andrea underwent a procedure to improve upon the scar and reported feeling happier with her appearance. She stated that a third factor impacting her mood was witnessing her father have a psychotic break and require hospitalization when she was 8 years old. She reported that, prior to age 8, both of her parents were well treated with medications and seemed

> …completely normal to me, just like the parents of any of my neighborhood friends. I would have otherwise had no idea, possibly ever, that either of them had any psychiatric issues. My mother was somewhat quiet and my father was a bit unemotional, but I never thought that either had any psychiatric problems. I had what I think was a very good childhood with loving, protective parents, who worked their hardest to give me a normal, safe childhood. Then, over the course of a few weeks, my life changed forever, and I have not yet recovered. I remember it very clearly. I noticed that my father would come home from work and spend hours reading about surveillance in books and on the internet. While reading books and surfing the internet would be normal to many people, my father would usually just come home from work and watch television and drink beer, so it was a noticeable change. He began to ignore us completely. He actually threw the television in the garbage and boarded up all of our windows. I did not realize it at the time, but he was extremely paranoid and developed persecutory delusions that the CIA was monitoring him and had hired an assassin to kill him. He stopped going to work, bought a gun, and was scared to go to sleep. This was the worst time of my life. My mother was very scared for my father as he was unwilling to take his medications or see his psychiatrist. He would spend all day on the couch next to our windows periodically, and stealthily, checking outside to see if anyone was outside. He was so preoccupied by his delusion that he stopped showering or shaving. He grew a short beard and smelled bad. For a few weeks as an 8-year-old I did not have a father. There was a stranger living in my home and I was scared of him.
>
> However, the worst was yet to come. My father began calling the police, asking them for protection from the "feds." They initially just ignored him. I am sure they receive calls like this every day. However, after several more calls, and as my father became more and more agitated and angry, the police decided to come to our apartment. I was there and will never forget what happened. The police came and my mother let them into the apartment.

However, when my father saw them, despite that they showed their badges and he had called them, he was convinced that they were acting on behalf of the CIA and were planning to kill him. He yelled "they found me!" and lunged for one of the officer's guns. He would have had it, except that, fortunately, the other officer was quick to react and put my father in a headlock. The other officer quickly regained his footing and helped to take down my father who was, in his mind, fighting for his life. My father was a large, strong man to begin with, and on this day he was so scared that he must have had superhuman strength. The police officers called for backup and before long six additional officers had come to our home and helped to subdue my father. All the time he was screaming and yelling that the CIA and police were going to kill him. He kept looking at me and my mother begging for us to not let them take him away to be murdered. My mother and I were scared and crying. I did not know what was going on but was permanently traumatized. My mother kept telling the police that my father has schizoaffective disorder and had not been taking his medications. She was also severely affected and traumatized by this. She looked so helpless and sad at that moment.

Eventually, an ambulance arrived and my father was taken to an emergency room. My mother asked one of our neighbors to look after me that evening while she went to the emergency room. The rest of that evening is a blur. All I remember is how my whole world felt like it had been turned upside down. Up until that time I, like most children, thought that my father was my hero, perfect and infallible. I felt that I was always safe when he was around. Whenever I was sad he was there to make me feel better. All he had to do was hug me and tell me everything was going to be alright, and I would immediately feel better. Now, I had just seen my father in an incredibly vulnerable state, acting less like a hero and more like a person who had completely lost his sanity. My world had crumbled and I began to realize that my idyllic, innocent, child-like view of life had forever been shattered.

The next time that I saw my father was five weeks later when he came home from the hospital. My mother refused to allow me or my sister to visit him while he was in the hospital. I realize now that she wanted to do her best to shelter us from their psychiatric illness and allow us to lead as normal lives as possible. My feelings upon seeing my father again were mixed. Of course I was very happy to see him, but was unsure how to act around him and was unsure of whether he was still preoccupied with the CIA or other persecutory delusions and whether he would remember me. Of course, he did remember me and my sister and was very happy to see us. For the most part he seemed the way that I had remembered him, although he did move a little more slowly. Fortunately, he was able to resume his job and, for the most part, life went back to normal. My sister and I spent time with our friends and at school. Both of us went to high school and attended our proms. My mother and father continued to work. Their relationship remained strong. From the outside, one could say that my childhood, with the exception of the time around my father's psychotic episode, was quite normal, just like any other.

And it was. I really have no right to complain about my childhood. I had loving parents. We were solidly in the middle class and never had to worry about food, clothing, or shelter, while many of my friends at school did have to worry about these things. Some of my friends even had parents in jail or prison. I felt very sorry for them and always remembered how lucky I was to have parents who were available to me. In addition, we were otherwise very healthy. My mother had acromegaly and looked a little different than other parents, but has not had any serious medical complications. We were even able to take yearly vacations, usually to some beach town in Maryland or Virginia.

There was only one thing that was different. I never forgot what happened to my father when he had his psychotic relapse and, even at the best of times, could not shake the fear that my father would have another. I became hypervigilant about his behavior. Any time he became even a little upset or showed emotion (compared to his usual which was relatively emotionless), I would remember the emotion that he showed when he was concerned about the CIA and I would begin to worry that he was becoming psychotic again. One time, while I was in my bed, I heard police sirens approach my building followed by police walking through the hall on my floor and thought, for a moment, that they may be coming for my father. I remember another time when I was in my room playing with my friend that I heard something vague, coming from our living room, about a CIA operation. I went to see what this was and found that my parents were watching a documentary on political espionage. My most upsetting nightmares involve situations in which my father becomes psychotic. It always takes at least 24 hours for me to get over these nightmares. Suffice it to say that I have never been able to rid myself of the background fear that, at any moment, my father may become psychotic again. Nothing in the world scares me more than this possibility.

[Andrea began to choke up and almost let down a tear, clearly feeling emotional about discussing these feelings, then quickly recovered.] Either way, everything was fine. My father never again spoke about the CIA nor became psychotic. I made my way through school, graduated high school, and went to college. My sister also finished high school and is now in college, though she went as far away as possible for college, to California, I think to escape the memories that she and I share. Laura loves our parents as much as, or even more than, I do, but I think was even more affected by what happened to our father than I was, because she was younger. Out of sight, out of mind, right? Anyway, as I was saying, everything turned out fine.

My parents have remained stable for over a decade and are only a few years away from retirement. My sister and I are in college. I will be graduating in four months and have already found a job with a consulting firm. However, most importantly, and the reason I am here, is because I just became engaged to my boyfriend, "Daniel." He is a wonderful person – kind, thoughtful, modest, and hard working. He will be entering dental school in the Fall. We met in our freshman economics class and hit it off immediately. We have been inseparable since. We have no set timetable for our marriage, but both know that we want to have at least two children. This will likely not happen before two to three years from now because Daniel will need to focus on dental school and I will have to focus on my job. However, with all these great things happening, I have developed anxiety about our relationship. It is not that I have any doubts about Daniel. On the contrary, there is no doubt that Daniel is the right person for me and I for him. We are committed to each other in every way. My anxiety is about having children. I am not sure that broken people like me should be having children. I love my parents more than anything else and know that they gave me the best life that I could have ever had. At the same time, I would never, ever, want my children to go through what I had to go through, worrying that their parents may become psychotic; never being able to fully relax. I think that people who have parents who are not psychotic could never understand how difficult it is to worry about their parents literally losing their mind. I know that my chances of developing schizophrenia are high, especially since I have two psychotic parents. And believe me, I am very scared of developing schizophrenia. But even worse is the thought that I could have children who would have to go through what I went through. I would rather not have kids than bring children into this world who have to deal with having a psychotic parent. Even worse would be passing along my genes to them and having to watch as they develop schizophrenia. I would never forgive myself.

Additionally, I would not want to do this to Daniel. He is the love of my life, but it would not be fair for him to have to deal with me if I were to become psychotic. I love him too much for that. He is well aware of my parents' conditions and what I went through as a child. He always tells me that he is not worried and does not care about any of that. He is very sweet and loving, and I fully believe him. However, I don't know if he could ever truly understand how bad it could be. And that is why I am here. I know that I am at high-risk for developing schizophrenia. Not only do both of my parents have schizophrenia, but, over the last year, I have experienced a number of disturbing symptoms. For example, for three months I have had the experience that my world is not real. The feeling is vague and I cannot describe it further, but it is somewhat bothersome. I have also been experiencing déjà vu. I know that déjà vu experiences are not uncommon, but, given everything else that has been going on, and that my parents have schizophrenia, I thought it would be good to speak to a psychiatrist about these experiences.

For about two years I have had the very odd feeling that things that I watch on television are referring to me. For example, yesterday I was watching a television program about a series of unsolved murders. Law enforcement were explaining why they thought that the unidentified suspect, who was determined to be male, most likely had a female accomplice. I know this sounds strange, but I had the sense that they were suggesting that I am involved in criminal activity and that they were coming for me. Further, about two years ago, for approximately six months, I thought that I was emitting an odor similar to that of rancid peanut butter from my mouth. I began to chew gum almost constantly while around people and would brush my teeth and use mouthwash five times a day. I also avoided Daniel. He reassured me that there was no odor coming from my mouth and I would believe him for the time being, then begin to doubt again a few hours later. Fortunately, this thought simply resolved itself within a few months, but it was concerning.

For three years I have had the daily sense that people might be judging or thinking negatively of me. This has increased in the past year, leading to a vague sense of being scorned by people. I think that they can tell that I have family members with schizophrenia and want to emotionally harm me. In addition, I have occasionally felt that people are staring at me trying to figure out how I came to have a scar on my face and wondering whether this means that I am a bad or dangerous person, one whom they might not like to befriend. Last summer, I had an incident of feeling that three men at my summer internship were coming too close to me, making me worry that they might wish to attack me.

I know inside of me that I have an average intelligence, but for some reason I have been thinking that people generally find me to be very intelligent, like a savant, and therefore different than them. In fact, I have noticed signs that I may become very powerful, but then I come back to reality and remind myself that this is not logical, nor do I want this. I would rather be anonymous and just have a plain, uneventful, happy life with Daniel and two or three children.

Sometimes I hear music or sounds, like humming or bumblebees. I occasionally hear what sounds like a cough saying my name. Several days ago I thought I saw a shadowy figure in the hallway that resembled Daniel. It startled me. It turned out to be a bunch of suits that were hanging on a door.

Because of Andrea's attenuated positive symptoms, as well as her family history, she was at high-risk for developing schizophrenia. While the risk of developing schizophrenia is approximately 9% in people with one parent with schizophrenia, that risk increases substantially to ~35%–40% when one has two family members with schizophrenia, as did Andrea (1).

As described by Andrea, individuals with an affected relative, especially a parent with schizophrenia, have many challenges that they need to face. These include: 1) the trauma of watching a parent act in a psychotic way; 2) the anxiety related to constantly worrying about the parent relapsing and having no control over this; 3) the fear of developing schizophrenia oneself, and the potential effect this would have on one's own family; and 4) the worry about passing on a genetic susceptibility to schizophrenia.

During Andrea's two years in our clinic we spent much of her time in therapy dealing with these issues through both psychoeducation and an insight-oriented psychotherapy in which we explored her experiences and feelings, their motivations, and how they had affected her life. First, we affirmed the traumatizing nature of having a psychotic parent, including the constant fear of relapse. Few experiences are as traumatizing and frightening to children. The feelings of hopelessness, depression, vulnerability, anxiety, lack of confidence, and stigma are real and can be compared to the severe stress of adults when they are forced to have a stoma. Few experiences are as emotionally challenging and harsh as having a psychotic parent.

We also dealt with Andrea's concerns about developing schizophrenia herself and the potential effects on Daniel and her family. We explored her own feelings about having grown up in a family with two psychotic parents and helped her to understand that, despite her parents' diagnoses, she grew up in a healthy, happy, loving household, had an otherwise supportive and nurturing childhood, and had happy parents who themselves would have changed nothing. We educated Andrea about her actual chances of developing a psychotic illness. She took particular solace knowing that, after two years in our clinic, if she had not yet developed a psychotic condition, the chances that she would develop one would be very low.

Finally, we explored Andrea's feelings about passing on "tainted" genetic material, even if she were not to develop schizophrenia. During her time in our clinic she learned that, even though psychiatric conditions, especially schizophrenia, are very biological and genetically determined, the majority of people with schizophrenia do not have family members with schizophrenia. These cases may be more related to de novo genetic abnormalities or other etiologies. We explained that, for example, if schizophrenia were completely genetic and familial in the way that most people understand heritability, then an identical twin of someone with schizophrenia would almost definitely develop schizophrenia, whereas in reality the risk of developing schizophrenia when one has an identical twin with schizophrenia is less than 50% (1).

Andrea responded very well to psychotherapy. At no time during her treatment with us did she require medications. Her mood remained good and her anxiety was low. Andrea eventually did graduate from college and began working at a consulting firm. Her fiancé, Daniel, matriculated at dental school. He was, per

Andrea's report, doing well and enjoying his chosen field. Andrea's sister continued at college in California and enjoyed her time there. Andrea's parents remained on their medications and were months away from retirement.

Over time, Andrea's attenuated positive symptoms began to remit. She no longer had grandiose ideas, referential thinking, or unusual perceptual experiences. She rarely thought that people were thinking negatively of her. By all measures, it appeared that Andrea was likely to be among the 70% in our high-risk clinic who was not going to convert.

Despite Andrea's progress in terms of both symptom remission and the work she had done in therapy to come to terms with her concerns, we could tell that she would not allow herself to move on with her life until the two year mark, after which her risk of developing a psychotic disorder would be extremely small.

That time came, shortly enough, when two years to the day that Andrea enrolled in our clinic, we met with her. She was noticeably happy and energetic. She told us that she and Daniel had set a date for their wedding. She told us that she had learned that schizophrenia, though a terrible and devastating disease, is no different than any other chronic disease, and that, regardless of what happens, she had come to terms with her situation and would deal with it. She reported that she had developed a new love for, and appreciation of, her parents and was determined to take a more active role in their treatment and care, especially as they became older. She also explained that she had several conversations with her sister and was helping her to begin to deal with the trauma that she also experienced as a child.

We continued to see Andrea for several years thereafter, through her marriage, her parents' retirement, and the birth of her first child. She remained fully remitted and never displayed any further psychotic symptoms, attenuated or otherwise. Her sister came back to the East Coast to be close to the family. Andrea's parents remained remitted and found new joy in their lives spending time with their daughters and grandchild, who was named "Wilson."

Reference

1.   McGue M, Gottesman, II. Genetic linkage in schizophrenia: perspectives from genetic epidemiology. *Schizophr Bull.* 1989;15(3):453–464.

4

THE FIRST-EPISODE OF PSYCHOSIS AND SUICIDE IN SCHIZOPHRENIA

"A." was a 25-year-old Asian bisexual female. She lived with her 63-year-old father, a stockbroker, 60-year-old stay-at-home mother, and 16-year-old sister, who was in high school. She reported positive relationships with all her family members.

A. described herself as "social" in childhood, with diminished interest in connecting with other people due to the onset of agoraphobia symptoms in the ninth grade. She stated that, while in nursing school and before she developed schizophrenia, she had four close friends whom she would see almost daily. She reported that she still kept in touch with these friends via email, but rarely saw them in person. She had never been married and had no children. She had never been in a romantic relationship, but was "sort of" interested in having one in the future.

A. reported earning "very good" grades across her academic career, until reaching nursing school. She developed schizophrenia during her first year of nursing school at a prestigious institution, requiring her to drop out. She had graduated at the top of her class in college and spent a year between college and nursing school in Zimbabwe providing HIV protection education to village populations. By all accounts, A. had performed very well in her first semester of nursing school. During the second semester she began to develop a delusion that her roommate's Pomeranian, along with several of the patient's nursing school colleagues, was plotting to kill her. A. was hospitalized late in her first year of nursing school and never made a full recovery. She began to develop impairments in cognition, such as attention, memory, and concentration, that precluded her from performing well in nursing school. She eventually took a medical leave of absence, and then dropped out of nursing school altogether.

Dropping out of nursing school was a severe blow to A.'s self-esteem, from which she had not recovered. Over the next 18 months she was admitted to psychiatric hospitals twice and was unable to return to nursing school. An ongoing theme in her therapy sessions was her feelings of regret and poor self-worth related to being unable to continue or complete nursing school. These sorts of feelings are unfortunately common in individuals shortly after their first episode of psychosis, especially when patients recover and begin to realize how great of an effect the diagnosis of schizophrenia can have on their lives. Although approximately 10%–20% can expect a relatively full recovery, many individuals have substantial functional impairment for the rest of their lives or require chronic care or institutionalization (1). Almost 5% commit suicide (2). A. was very aware of these facts as she had learned about schizophrenia in nursing school. She was also aware that suicide in schizophrenia is particularly common during the first- and early-episode time periods, for the reasons described above, and while these individuals have a preserved affect and ability to experience the full range of emotions (3).

At the time of her hospitalization at our institution, A. was working part-time as a nanny, ten hours per week. She described the work as "boring." She described her mood as "Blah." She had a constricted affect, and slow, monotone, and occasionally mumbled speech. Her degree of spontaneous conversation was within normal limits. She sometimes exhibited inappropriate smiling and giggling. Some occasional fidgeting was noted. At several points in the evaluation she sat in an odd, crouched position on the chair. A. reported an extensive history of odd obsessions and compulsions since childhood. While A. described some dysphoria in early adolescence due to frustration with obsessive-compulsive symptoms, she denied any significant history of depressive or manic symptoms, or irritability, and none were evident. She denied any past or current suicidal, self-injurious or violent ideation, plan, intent, or behaviors, or access to weapons. She had never been arrested.

A. denied any history of psychiatric treatment prior to age 15 when she visited a private psychiatrist who diagnosed her with depression and obsessive-compulsive disorder. As a senior in college she saw a school counselor for anxiety.

Upon admission to our hospital, A. reported and/or displayed a number of positive symptoms. She reported the sense that she had the ability to control nature, for example, by controlling bacteria, viruses, and other microorganisms. She explained that if someone were to become infected, she could heal them. She similarly reported that she could infect someone at will, "but would never do something like that." When asked how she had control of microorganisms, she explained that she had developed this ability by learning how to communicate and "become one" with her own bodily flora. She reported that she had no choice but to gain this ability because the microorganisms that were inhabiting her own body (her own bodily flora) were trying to take control of her body and so she had no choice but to learn how to control and communicate with them. A. went on to say that another reason she had to learn how to control them was that she was concerned that the microorganisms in her own body would seek out other people and try to infect them. When A. began having these thoughts, she would do everything she could to prevent infecting other people, such as by wearing masks, hats, and multiple layers of long sleeve shirts and long pants whenever she went outside, including on days when the weather was very warm. She also began surreptitiously taking antibiotics that she would steal from outpatient clinics and inpatient units at the hospital affiliated with her nursing school. A. would go through an eight-ounce bottle of hand sanitizer every day and spend at least an hour a day washing her hands. Her showers would take 45 minutes. A.'s life became much easier once she learned to take control of her bodily flora.

A. reported that there were a few people who were colonized, but not infected, by her flora. A. was unable to prevent the microbial flora from colonizing these people, but was able to learn how to control the microorganisms in time to protect these people from infection. The three people were a classmate in nursing school, her neighbor's 18-month-old son, and her own gynecologist "Dr. Luca." The classmate in nursing school was a lady named "Theodora." A. and Theodora sat a row apart during nursing school lectures. Theodora was the smartest person in A.'s nursing school class and obtained the highest grades on all their exams. A. was attracted to Theodora, but had to avoid Theodora to prevent her infestation and colonization.

The 18-month-old son of A.'s neighbor was named "Campbell." Campbell's father was an attorney who worked for a major law firm. Campbell's mother was a dermatologist. A. would occasionally babysit Campbell when she was visiting home from nursing school. A. felt guilty that her microorganisms had colonized young Campbell, but was happy to have been able to prevent his infection.

Dr. Luca was A.'s gynecologist. A. did not like Dr. Luca. She felt that Dr. Luca had a terrible bedside manner and was superficial, arrogant, and fake. Dr. Luca would regularly try to persuade A. to take opioid medications for minor discomfort. A. continued to see Dr. Luca because he was a graduate of one of the top OB-GYN departments in the country. A. was not sorry that he was colonized.

A. presented as somewhat expansive at times. She described a sense that her ability to communicate with and control microorganisms was "godlike." She denied being a god, but just that she had, out of necessity, developed a skill that no human could ever have or would have again. She described herself as being "no different than leading scientists, but in a metaphysical sense." She would occasionally joke that she could have won the Nobel Prize if she had "put my mind to it."

A. did not present as guarded. She reported vague suspicious thoughts that someone, such as the daytime doorman at her building, might wish to kidnap her. This prompted A. to either avoid going out during the day or use a side entrance. A. was also generally careful around people she did not otherwise know. However, she denied any past or current sense that she should prepare to defend herself or arm herself related to suspicious thoughts.

A. did not appear internally preoccupied at any point during the evaluation process. She reported occasionally seeing shadows in the corner of her eye across her lifetime, but no formed images. She also described instances, across her lifetime, of feeling a warm or tingly sensation on her body or smelling something others did not, which prompted thoughts that she might have been feeling or reading other people's energies or auras, but never paid much attention to them. She denied perceptual abnormalities in any other sensory modality. When asked about whether or not she heard sounds or voices when communicating with the microorganisms, she laughed and said, "That is silly. What medical school did you go to? Viruses and single-celled organisms are too simple to communicate with language. My connection with them is more like how mediums speak with the deceased."

A. was notably vague, circumstantial, and occasionally tangential. She usually responded to redirection. Her associations were not uncommonly loose. She admitted that, since developing schizophrenia, people had been telling her that she had become more difficult to follow. Further, in the previous year, she had noticed that, several times per day, she would lose her train of thought in conversations, or when attempting to follow directions or complete assignments.

It was late on a Wednesday evening. We had finished seeing our last outpatients of the day and were heading home. We were at the elevator when we heard a call for a medical emergency on the overhead announcement system.

There is an important difference between medical emergencies in medical versus psychiatric hospitals. In medical hospitals, an emergency that is announced overhead generally indicates that a patient is in impending or imminent cardiac or respiratory arrest, or that the patient has already arrested. Medical staff are generally extremely responsive to such calls, and within seconds of an emergency call, one would typically observe between 15–20 nurses and physicians in an all-out sprint to the patient's room.

Medical emergencies in psychiatric hospitals are very different. They are most often called for episodes of fainting, or dizziness, and rarely for true medical emergencies. There is a joke among mental health clinicians that a nosebleed would be considered a medical emergency at some psychiatric hospitals. Most staff at psychiatric hospitals understand this fact and, therefore, when a medical emergency is called at a psychiatric hospital, one usually does not observe the rush of tens of medical staff toward a patient's room, but rather a few individuals running to get to the patient's room, and then 10–15 more walking at a somewhat robust pace.

This evening was no different. After the medical emergency was called, we did not observe a single person making their way to the inpatient unit. Although not close to the unit, we sprinted to the unit as quickly as possible and let ourselves onto the unit. There was a notable dearth of medical staff on the unit. One nurse was frantically calling somebody. When she saw us, she pointed toward the storage room, apparently indicating where the emergency was.

We ran into the storage room and found the patient huddled in the corner. She had pierced her left abdomen, around her spleen, with a hanger, which was now on the floor, while the patient, apparently having punctured an artery, was profusely bleeding.

One of us immediately was given a towel that a female nurse (who had accompanied us into the room) had seized and pressed it into the patient's spleen area to stop the heavy bleeding while the patient was fighting us off. The other ran to gather more staff to help restrain the patient. While struggling with A. to prevent her from further movement, she would scream that she wanted to die. She pleaded with us to allow her to kill herself. Shortly thereafter, additional staff came and helped to restrain the patient. She required manual restraints and several rounds of intramuscular medications in order to calm down, which she eventually did, while she was being emergently transferred to the medical hospital for emergency surgery. Miraculously, she survived without any permanent damage, though was left with a moderately severe scar in the region of her spleen.

After being medically stabilized, A. returned to the psychiatric unit. Although not working on the inpatient unit ourselves, we were asked to assist with A.'s treatment, given how complicated she was. She was still delusional and disorganized. She also began to tell us more about her low mood, anergia, feelings of guilt, lack of interest in things in which she used to be interested, great desire to kill herself, poor appetite, and initial insomnia. In particular, A. stated that, if she had another opportunity to kill herself, she would take it "and would not mess up this time."

Because of how high-risk A. was (i.e., her great desire to kill herself), constant observation (aka, "1:1" or a "sitter"), at arms-length, was ordered for her. This means that, at all times, even when sleeping or using the restroom, A. was being observed by a staff member who was not just watching the patient, but was literally "at arms-length." This is required when patients are at particularly high risk of harming themselves, as was A. at the time.

Our next step was to develop a psychiatric treatment plan that would address both A.'s psychosis (i.e., her delusions about controlling microorganisms, disorganization, grandiosity, and paranoia), which had not responded to her current antipsychotic medication, risperidone, and her severe depression with suicidality. For this we decided on both psychotherapeutic and psychopharmacological interventions. For the medication intervention we considered many options, including other antipsychotic medications, antidepressants, and both. We knew we had to address her depression, psychosis, and suicidality. To address her lingering delusions and disorganization, we chose clozapine. Not only is clozapine the most effective antipsychotic medication, especially for treatment-refractory illness, but it is the only antipsychotic medication approved for recurrent suicidal behavior (4, 5). The reasons for its effectiveness against suicidal behavior and superior effectiveness for treatment-refractory psychosis are unknown. However, it was for these reasons that it was an optimal medication for A.

Given how severe A.'s situation was, we also wanted to directly treat her depression. For this we decided to add an antidepressant. In this case we chose fluoxetine.

Depression is common in psychotic individuals, especially during early episodes, and often requires co-treatment with antidepressant medications (6).

Finally, we implemented a psychotherapeutic intervention. We met with A. on a daily basis and worked through her substantial feelings of guilt, regret, shame, stigma, and hopelessness related to having been diagnosed with schizophrenia. We started by providing psychoeducation about living with schizophrenia, with a focus on how most people who develop schizophrenia receive treatment, are stable, and live normal or near-normal lives. We emphasized that media portrayals of schizophrenia overrepresent the violent, substance-using, treatment-refractory individuals who now make up a very small portion of the total population living with this condition.

After the psychoeducation component of the therapy we began to work with A. in a more insight-oriented manner, focusing on her own experiences, ideas, conflicts, and motivations. A. proved to be very psychologically minded and rapidly grew in the therapy. She began to understand how her own feelings about having schizophrenia, wanting to graduate nursing school and prove herself to be competent, and her envy of other people whom she viewed as more successful than she, were intertwined. For example, in one particularly effective session, A. responded very well to the interpretation that her delusions about controlling the microorganisms in the bodies of Theodora (the smartest person in her nursing school class), Dr. Luca (her gynecologist who was trained at one of the top programs in the country), and the 18-month-old son of her neighbor (who was a successful dermatologist) were in part an expression of her envy of these three successful clinicians or clinicians-to-be, a reflection of her own insecurities, and a desire to regain control or mastery of something, after having lost so much, in her mind, due to her schizophrenia.

This proved to be a watershed session for A. Within three days of this revelation A.'s depression had improved to such a great degree that she was transitioned from arm's length constant observation to normal constant observation, and then to 15-minute checks.

In addition, A. tolerated her medications well. She reached a clozapine dose of 200mg and a fluoxetine dose of 40mg. Her mood substantially improved and she was mostly free of delusions. She was fully linear and goal-directed. She began to socialize more on the unit. Within two weeks she was discharged, after having spent a total of eight weeks on the inpatient unit. Her wounds had completely healed.

A. continued to receive treatment at our outpatient clinic. Although she did not return to nursing school, she chose to pursue psychotherapy. She received a Master's degree in social work and went on to become a Licensed Clinical Social Worker. She joined a clinic for low-income patients as a psychotherapist. She felt very fulfilled by her work.

A. also made strides in her personal life. She met a lady in her social work program. They began dating while in school and eventually married and had two children. A. carried both children.

The last we heard from A. was three years ago when she stopped into our clinic to thank us for saving her life on the inpatient unit. She informed us that she was moving with her family to another part of the country and felt that she had been given a new opportunity in her life. She reported that she not only no longer regretted not becoming a nurse, but felt very happy that she left nursing school, as without having done so she would not have met her wife, had her children, and had the fulfilling life that she currently had.

References

1. Huber G. The heterogeneous course of schizophrenia. *Schizophr Res.* 1997;28(2–3):177–185.
2. Palmer BA, Pankratz VS, Bostwick JM. The lifetime risk of suicide in schizophrenia: a reexamination. *Arch Gen Psychiatry.* 2005;62(3):247–253.
3. Pompili M, Lester D, Grispini A, Innamorati M, Calandro F, Iliceto P, De Pisa E, Tatarelli R, Girardi P. Completed suicide in schizophrenia: evidence from a case-control study. *Psychiatry Res.* 2009;167(3):251–257.
4. Kane J, Honigfeld G, Singer J, Meltzer H. Clozapine for the treatment-resistant schizophrenic. A double-blind comparison with chlorpromazine. *Arch Gen Psychiatry.* 1988;45(9):789–796.
5. Meltzer HY, Alphs L, Green AI, Altamura AC, Anand R, Bertoldi A, Bourgeois M, Chouinard G, Islam MZ, Kane J, Krishnan R, Lindenmayer JP, Potkin S. Clozapine treatment for suicidality in schizophrenia: International Suicide Prevention Trial (InterSePT). *Arch Gen Psychiatry.* 2003;60(1):82–91.
6. Siris SG. Depression in schizophrenia: perspective in the era of "Atypical" anti-psychotic agents. *Am J Psychiatry.* 2000;157(9):1379–1389.

5

THE MANY CLINICAL PHASES
OF EARLY PSYCHOSIS
AND THE IMPORTANCE
OF PSYCHOEDUCATION AND
MEDICATION MANAGEMENT

In this chapter, we will describe one day of rounds on a psychiatric inpatient unit. We will describe four different patients with first-episode psychosis, each at a different phase of their hospitalization and their first episode, by which we will illustrate the dynamic and confusing nature of this phase of the illness, for patients and family alike. We will also use the interactions between the patients and the students on the unit to further describe this phase of the illness, with an emphasis on the importance of medications, psychoeducation, acute psychosis, stigma, the risk of relapse, and some of the differences between first-episode and chronic illness.

We entered the inpatient unit at 8:30am and reviewed our email. After the daily morning team meeting, during which the overnight nurses report on all the patients on the unit to the day team, we had a brief meeting with our specific team and began to see our patients.

The first patient of the day was "Max," a 24-year-old male who, around the age of 22 years old, became extremely paranoid about a certain cultural community. He thought that the members of this community were "trying to assimilate" other cultures, communities, and races with their genes and culture. He thought that this cultural group had the ability to control one's mind by looking through their eyes. As a result, he would avoid eye contact with anyone who looked or sounded like someone from this cultural community. Anytime he would leave the house he would wear sunglasses when there was a chance he would be around a person from this community. On the unit, where sunglasses were not allowed, and when a patient or staff who was potentially a member of this group would speak with him, he would address them but look away, such as at the ceiling or to the side. Max explained that, as long as one did not look at these people, they could do no harm.

This delusion was confusing at first because Max was a member of this cultural community, as was his family. His whole family was, apparently, exempt from his delusions. Max had revealed, in the course of his treatment on the unit, that, when Max was very young, his family was ostracized from the community for not adhering to a certain tradition. Therefore, although Max's family identified with this group, they were considered outsiders and non-adherents.

As Max's psychosis worsened, he became involved with a number of hate groups whose rhetoric was focused on his own community. He adopted their dress, tattooed their symbol on his arm, and was constantly spouting paranoid vitriol at people, including strangers.

What complicated matters was that he was also struggling with a developing gay sexual identity and could not reconcile his beliefs with the fact that he had relationships with men in the past, including with a partner from his own community. He had intense paranoid ideas surrounding people finding this out by hacking into his computer and reading his email messages or searching through his internet history and finding that he had been frequenting gay dating sites. Sometimes he heard voices calling him derogatory terms for people who belong to his community.

Max was originally brought to the emergency room by his parents when they found him writing a manifesto online about how it was his duty to rid the Earth of this group of people for their desire to assimilate other cultures, communities, and races. They had also found several weapons, including semi-automatic guns, knives, and a crossbow in Max's bedroom.

On the unit Max was calm and mostly cooperative, besides that he insisted that no one among his treatment team be a member of his community. However, there was a student on the unit who was a member of his community and whom Max avoided at great length. In his daily therapy sessions, Max would frequently ask for information about the student, such as her background, whether we were worried she might try to assimilate us, and whether she had told us about her plan to assimilate him, or potentially just kill him for being attracted to men.

Max responded very well to low doses of loxipane, as individuals in the first-episode of psychosis tend to do. Sometimes 80% or more of individuals with first-episode psychosis respond to antipsychotic medications (1), hence one of the main reasons why beginning antipsychotic medications is so important, especially early in one's illness. While patients with chronic schizophrenia also respond well to antipsychotic medications, they tend to have lower response rates (2). The antipsychotic medications that are considered "first-line" in first-episode psychosis are typically second-generation medications besides clozapine and olanzapine (3). It is felt that these medications balance efficacy with side effects.

Psychosocial treatments, such as counseling or psychotherapy, are also a very important part of treatment in first-episode psychosis. Patients who are early in their illness may often have sustained insight, or simply less negative symptoms and cognitive deficits, than someone later in their illness, allowing a relatively more insight-oriented dynamic approach to therapy than a fully supportive dynamic approach that might be more appropriate for a patient in later stages of the illness.

Once the medications began to take effect and the strength of Max's delusions subsided, Max proved to be very amenable to an insight-oriented therapy and generally psychologically minded. Max responded well to the observation that his delusions could be considered a response to the years of exclusion and stigma imposed upon Max by his own community – feelings that he had internalized. The therapy also helped Max come to terms with his sexual identity. He began to realize that, although his community was not accepting of his lifestyle, his family was very supportive and did not care what their community would think of them for Max being gay.

Ultimately, Max did very well. He was discharged within three days. He made a nearly full recovery and continued in a weekly therapy. His family remained very supportive of him and his sexual preferences. He continued his medications and, as of the writing of this book, had not required rehospitalization.

The next patient we saw was "Wendy," a 19-year-old female from an upper-middle-class family from New Jersey. She had two siblings and what could be described as a "typical" upbringing. Her father, "Thomas," was a chemical engineer and her mother, "Diane," was a homemaker. The family would go to a Presbyterian church every Sunday, followed by a brunch at a local diner. They had two cars, a dog named "Miss Sadie," and a cat named "Fluffy." Every year they would take two vacations, one in the Summer to the Jersey Shore and another in the winter to either Florida or the Southwestern United States. Wendy's father played on a corporate softball team and her mother was on the high school's parent teacher association. They lived in a neighborhood in which there were only three different house designs and so every third house looked alike, with slight differences in color. Wendy's older brother, "Charlie," played college baseball. Wendy's younger brother, "Corey," played high school football.

We saw Wendy on her first day on the unit, a few hours after she had been transferred from the emergency room. According to the emergency room sign out, Wendy was brought to the emergency room after she was found yelling at the food service workers in her college dormitory, accusing them of trying to poison her.

We met with Wendy and her parents who had come to the hospital when they heard that Wendy had been sent to the emergency room. Wendy was a well-dressed, young female, approximately five feet, five inches tall with blonde hair in a messy bun. She had light makeup on. She was pleasant and spoke in a "Valleyspeak" accent. She asked for access to her smartphone numerous times. She was organized and had a good mood, though did admit to being, and appeared to be, frustrated with being on a psychiatric inpatient unit.

Wendy and her family further explained Wendy's behavior over the previous few months. Wendy had been doing well until just before she began college, three months previous. She broke up with her high school boyfriend of two years and said that he was an "evil" person. The family attributed her behavior and what she was saying to having just broken up with her boyfriend and did not pay much attention to it. In college, Wendy was able to pass her classes, but did have a hard time making friends. She would report to her parents that nobody liked her and she spent most of her time in her dormitory room. Again, the parents figured that she was simply struggling with adapting to college and paid little attention to what was happening.

On the unit, Wendy clarified that she felt that, over the previous several months, people were jealous of her and therefore targeting her. For example, her boyfriend was jealous that she was going to a better college than he was and began cheating on her. At school, many of the students and service workers were jealous of her because she had more money than they did. They began saying derogatory things about her, such as that she is "ugly," "stupid," and a "slut." She would often hear people come up to her window and yell things at her, or yell from her neighbors' rooms. Wendy became very upset the previous day and yelled at one of the food service workers whom she thought was trying to poison her food.

Wendy had no apparent negative symptoms or cognitive deficits. Her mood was euthymic. She was organized and attentive, albeit delusional and experiencing hallucinations (though not during the interview). Wendy had no medical problems and her family history was negative for any psychiatric illness, outside of "crazy uncle Joe" whom the family said had received a diagnosis of schizophrenia when he was 20 years old, but was really just "morally confused" and a "junkie" according to Wendy's parents. Wendy denied using any substances and reported that she had only been drunk twice in her life. Her urine toxicology was negative.

We diagnosed Wendy with first-episode psychosis, likely schizophrenia, and recommended medication management as well as psychotherapy. We spent a great deal of time educating the patient and her family about psychosis, including what it is (i.e., the symptoms), the treatment options and importance of early treatment with medications, the course of the illness including the high risk of relapse when not taking medications, the problem of insight, side effects of medications, and prognosis. Wendy and her parents listened with great interest and intent. They asked questions that showed that they were listening closely and really wanted to learn from and understand what we were saying. Toward the end of the session, the mother asked if Wendy had schizophrenia, to which we replied:

Dr. Girgis: It does appear that Wendy has developed a psychotic disorder. It is very possible that this could be schizophrenia, although we will not know for sure until we spend a little more time with Wendy and obtain more information on the course of her illness going forward.

Diane: Thank you doctor. We are really grateful for the great help and care you have shown to our daughter Wendy, whom we love beyond what you could imagine. Of note, I was reading online about bipolar disorder and, to me, not being an expert, it seems like she is much more likely to have bipolar disorder.

We cannot count the number of times we have had this exact same discussion with patients and their families. Understandably, they read online about mental illness. First, they read about schizophrenia and psychosis and how it is a chronic illness. Their viewpoint is greatly shaped by the public's view of schizophrenia, which is one of intractable symptoms and inexorable mental deterioration born from images of the homeless, media depictions of psychotic killers, and the entertainment industry's exploitation of mental illness for dramatic purposes. They are not aware of the research over the last three decades that has provided evidence of the effectiveness of treatment that may change the course and even prevent the onset of the illness. Families then read about bipolar disorder, anxiety, and depression which, though stigmatized, do not carry near the same negative valence as does schizophrenia. People read about how many very successful, rich, attractive, and powerful people have these conditions and so they allow themselves to ignore their family member's symptoms due to shame, stigma, miseducation, or other personal reasons. This does not happen all of the time, but definitely happens most of the time when we see patients in the early stages of their illness while patients and families are most vulnerable and still coming to terms with, learning about, and trying to understand what is happening to their affected family member. We cannot blame anyone for preferring to carry a diagnosis of an anxiety or mood disorder to a psychotic disorder. That is one of the main reasons we are writing this book – to disabuse clinicians and lay people of the therapeutic nihilism and stigma that have historically pervaded the field.

We spent hours with Wendy and her parents, providing greater education and doing our best to help them understand that a diagnosis of schizophrenia is not a death sentence for the majority of people. Rather, schizophrenia, especially in its earlier stages, is extremely responsive to treatment and the chances were strongly in Wendy's favor that, as long as she continued in treatment, she could have led a very normal life.

Unfortunately, despite our greatest efforts, including demonstrating that Wendy met no criteria for bipolar disorder, mania, or depression, it did not appear that Wendy or her family were able to accept her diagnosis. They were very pleasant, thanked us profusely for our time and care, and then asked for Wendy to be discharged home, after which they would have her see their primary care physician whom they had known for 20 years, for a full consultation.

We were beginning to see our next patient when another patient with first-episode psychosis, "Paul," an 18-year-old male, became acutely psychotic and agitated. He had been admitted to the inpatient unit the night before after being found on the street with a cape on his back, claiming to be a superhero, saying that he needed to save the city from his archenemy. He had required several rounds of intramuscular medications the night before and had slept through the morning. While individuals with schizophrenia can at times be severely agitated and uncontrollable, this often occurs in the context of substance-induced psychosis or mania. Paul had not been using street drugs. However, as we later learned, Paul actually had schizoaffective disorder. Schizoaffective disorder is very closely related to schizophrenia. People with schizoaffective disorder meet all of the same criteria as do people with schizophrenia, except that they also have a number of other features, including: 1) having at least one major mood episode (mania or major depressive episode) during their illness; 2) having delusions or hallucinations for at least two weeks without a major mood episode; and 3) having symptoms that meet criteria for a major mood episode that last for a majority of the condition (4). People with schizoaffective disorder also tend to have few negative symptoms and less functional impairment (5, 6). Their prognosis is somewhat better than what it is for people with schizophrenia and somewhat worse than what it is for people with purely affective disorders, such as major depressive disorder or bipolar disorder.

Paul had several weeks of delusions and hallucinations related to being a superhero and hearing the voice of his archenemy, then had a month of a full manic episode with severe irritability, decreased need for sleep, increased energy, impulsiveness, racing thoughts, fast speech, and grandiosity. Therefore, Paul was experiencing a psychotic mania in the context of schizoaffective disorder. Individuals experiencing a psychotic mania can be very aggressive, impulsive, and dangerous, and require very close and attentive management, as well as aggressive treatment with medications.

Paul had apparently just awakened from sleep, jumped the security guard who was outside of his room, and ran toward the door screaming that his archenemy was going to poison the city's air supply if he did not do something about it. We called a hospital-wide psychiatric emergency and, with the help of a quickly mobilized team of security, mental health aides, and nurses who were on the unit, were able to take down Paul and place him in a quiet room. The situation was under control and no one had been injured. Then, as one of the nurses was injecting Paul with intramuscular medications, a mental health aide suddenly yelled, "Oh no! Who is watching the eating disorder patients?!"

Eating disorder patients, such as those with bulimia and anorexia nervosa, follow very strict meal and diet protocols, given their propensity for restriction, binging, purging, and excessive exercise. In addition to following very detailed and strict diets, they are monitored during all their meals and for one hour afterwards to ensure that they eat all their food and do not vomit their food. On this day, Paul became agitated right after the patients had finished their lunch. They were all in a television room during their period of post-lunch monitoring. When Paul became severely agitated and the emergency was called, seeing that there were not enough people on the unit, the mental health aide who was responsible for monitoring the eating disorder patients reflexively, and appropriately, ran to help manage Paul. Free from their monitor, the eating disorder patients covertly went to their rooms and bathrooms and all vomited up their lunch.

Fortunately, Paul was safe and, after several more days of medications and close monitoring, recovered from his psychotic mania. The eating disorder patients also resumed their normal protocol without further interruption.

Our last patient on rounds was "Herbert," a 25-year-old married Korean male who worked as a doorman. He had been psychotic over a period of 18 months, following a 12-month prodrome. He had immigrated to America with his wife only four years prior. His initial prodromal, attenuated positive symptoms included a vague sense that people were following him, as well as that his 5-month-old infant was possessed by the devil. He reported 60% conviction about both thoughts and did not allow them to affect his functioning. He was able to continue to work and care for his family. He also reported seeing shadows in the corner of his eye, twice weekly, during his prodromal period. He indicated that, once a week, he had the idea that he was destined to become famous, or already was famous, because of how people would look at him. Herbert retained insight during the first ten months of his prodromal period and sought out treatment from a psychiatrist in the community who appropriately initially treated the patient with an anti-depressant and then with an antipsychotic medication. Unfortunately, Herbert's symptoms progressed. During the last two months of his prodromal period, his visual perceptual abnormalities resolved, but his ideas that his infant son was possessed by the devil, and that people were following him, achieved 100% con-viction. Herbert reported that he began to realize that his son, who was possessed by the devil, had mobilized legions of demons to follow him and, eventually, murder him. The devil wanted to kill Herbert because he was a messenger from God. Herbert knew this because he began to hear God giving him instructions on whom to save and whom to condemn.

As a consequence of these delusions and hallucinations, Herbert began staying away from his home, throwing holy water on his son, wrapping his son in garlic, and pressing Crucifixes onto his son's chest. He also began to miss work, thinking that his colleagues and boss had been possessed by evil spirits and were taking orders from his son.

Herbert had developed schizophrenia. He required several hospitalizations over the 18 months of his illness, usually because he would stop the medications that he was taking and which were treating his positive symptoms very well. When we saw him, Herbert was on his third hospitalization after having stopped risperidone for the third time and relapsing. We restarted the risperidone and had a discus-sion with Herbert and his family about long-acting, depot risperidone. Several antipsychotic medications, such as risperidone, haloperidol, and fluphenazine, come in long-acting, depot formulations, which are generally given as monthly or biweekly injections. They can be very effective for people who respond to anti-psychotic medications and have difficulties with adherence, like Herbert.

Herbert was very reluctant to take a long-acting medication given his generally impaired insight and fear of needles. Fortunately, in addition to the education and support that we provided, Herbert received a great deal of support and encouragement from "Tania," the social work student on our team. Tania spent a great deal of time with Herbert and his family. She was Korean American and was able to not only speak in their native Korean language, but provided Herbert with a level of trust and familiarity that he would not have otherwise been able to achieve with other members of the treatment team. Tania was also fully aware of the stigma of mental illness in Asian communities and allowed the family a safe place to speak about their feelings about Herbert's diagnosis, as well as their concerns about the future.

Herbert eventually agreed to begin long-acting risperidone and continued to recover. He experienced an almost complete resolution of his positive symptoms and demonstrated a level of insight that is not typically observed in individuals with schizophrenia. Unfortunately, over the course of Herbert's first-episode, he had also begun to develop negative symptoms and cognitive deficits. He was less emotive than usual. His wife felt less affection from Herbert than was typical for them. Herbert also demonstrated mild to moderate difficulties with attention and short-term memory. He seemed less interested in his hygiene than usual and began showering three to four times a week, rather than daily. He had also lost his job during the course of his first episode. Herbert's wife was very concerned about their finances since his was the only income. Tania was again instrumental in educating Herbert and his family about the realities of schizophrenia.

One of those realities is coordinated specialty care. Coordinated specialty care is a treatment for patients with first-episode psychosis (7, 8). It uses a recovery-based model with shared decision-making between specialists, the families, and their patients. Components of coordinated specialty care include medication management, psychotherapy/counseling, vocational training, case management, family education, and general support, all tailored toward a specific patient's needs and preferences. Coordinated specialty care has been implemented with great success in states such as New York (OnTrackNY) and will hopefully become widely implemented and the standard of care in the near future.

Since Herbert's symptoms had markedly improved, we began to prepare for his discharge. We had Herbert meet with a coordinated specialty care program at a local clinic. He and his family had a very positive experience with them and chose to continue their care with them. Herbert was discharged the next day, having been accepted to the clinic and stable on his medication.

References

1.   Robinson DG, Woerner MG, Alvir JM, Geisler S, Koreen A, Sheitman B, Chakos M, Mayerhoff D, Bilder R, Goldman R, Lieberman JA. Predictors of treatment response

from a first episode of schizophrenia or schizoaffective disorder. *Am J Psychiatry.* 1999;156(4):544–549.

2.   Sheitman BB, Lieberman JA. The natural history and pathophysiology of treatment resistant schizophrenia. *J Psychiatr Res.* 1998;32(3–4):143–150.

3.   Buchanan RW, Kreyenbuhl J, Kelly DL, Noel JM, Boggs DL, Fischer BA, Himelhoch S, Fang B, Peterson E, Aquino PR, Keller W. The 2009 schizophrenia PORT psychopharmacological treatment recommendations and summary statements. *Schizophr Bull.* 2009;36(1):71–93.

4.   American Psychiatric Association. *Diagnostic and statistical manual of mental disorders.* 5 ed. Washington, DC: American Psychiatric Association; 2013.

5.   Cheniaux E, Landeira-Fernandez J, Lessa Telles L, Lessa JL, Dias A, Duncan T, Versiani M. Does schizoaffective disorder really exist? A systematic review of the studies that compared schizoaffective disorder with schizophrenia or mood disorders. *J Affect Disord.* 2008;106(3):209–217.

6.   Mancuso SG, Morgan VA, Mitchell PB, Berk M, Young A, Castle DJ. A comparison of schizophrenia, schizoaffective disorder, and bipolar disorder: results from the Second Australian national psychosis survey. *J Affect Disord.* 2015;172:30–37.

7.   Dixon LB, Goldman HH, Bennett ME, Wang Y, McNamara KA, Mendon SJ, Goldstein AB, Choi CW, Lee RJ, Lieberman JA, Essock SM. Implementing coordinated specialty care for early psychosis: the RAISE Connection Program. *Psychiatr Serv.* 2015;66(7):691–698.

8.   Bello I, Lee R, Malinovsky I, Watkins L, Nossel I, Smith T, Ngo H, Birnbaum M, Marino L, Sederer LI, Radigan M, Gu G, Essock S, Dixon LB. OnTrackNY: the development of a coordinated specialty care program for individuals experiencing early psychosis. *Psychiatr Serv.* 2017;68(4):318–320.

PART II

Recurrent and Chronic Illness (Once You Have It How Do You Manage It)

6

DRUG-INDUCED AND OTHER ACUTE PSYCHOSES IN AN EMERGENCY-ROOM SETTING

The psychiatric emergency room is where a clinician will encounter some of the most acute, psychotic, and potentially dangerous patients – indeed, the mental health field's grueling front line. In this chapter, we will describe one of our most grueling and remarkable overnight calls in the psychiatric emergency room, allowing a discussion of several key topics, including medication-induced psychosis, severe agitation, treatment over objection, the safe management of acutely psychotic patients, and medical conditions that may mimic psychosis through several illustrative case histories.

Our psychiatric emergency room shift began at 11pm and was like any other shift. There were ten patients who had been seen during the day shift and were "tucked away" in emergency-room parlance, waiting for placement in psychiatric hospitals. Several patients were "on the board," which means waiting to be seen. We began right away, with Agatha.

"Agatha" was a 62-year-old African-American female with a history of mild anxiety. She was brought in by her husband, "Darrell," following several weeks of what he called "bizarre" behavior, which he described as "totally out of character" for her. He further explained that, just after they returned from a "second honeymoon" in Monte Carlo about a month prior, Agatha began complaining of mild back pain. Initially, Agatha and Darrell attributed this to having walked several miles daily and swimming a great deal while abroad. After a few days, however, Agatha's pain had progressed. Back in the United States, she saw her primary care physician who suggested a musculoskeletal issue and observed that Agatha appeared to him to be "a bit down," possibly because the couple's rare romantic getaway had come to an end. The physician prescribed lorazepam, a benzodiazepine, to help Agatha "take the edge off." Agatha started by taking 0.5mg lorazepam twice daily, quickly increasing to 1mg twice daily. She took this dose for two weeks. Unfortunately, her pain continued to grow. Additionally, Agatha began developing behavioral symptoms, such as speech that Darrell found vague and difficult to follow, staring into space, grasping at invisible things, and general confusion. At her worst, Agatha would start a sentence and fail to finish it. She also tended to spend much more time than usual in bed.

There was a diurnal variation to Agatha's symptoms. She tended to be relatively clear in the mornings, but was much more symptomatic after sundown. After several weeks of increasing symptoms, culminating one night when Agatha seemed particularly impaired, Darrell told his wife that he was concerned about her and wanted to take her to the emergency room. Agatha responded by slapping Darrell and accusing him of having always wanted to get rid of her. Darrell called 911 and an ambulance transported Agatha to a local ER.

Upon arrival, Agatha was screaming that Darrell wanted to have her "taken away" and that, after their long marriage, he was "tired" of her. She was occasionally grasping or swiping at objects that were not there. The previous attending physician, who did not have time to evaluate her at the end of his shift, wrote an order for 2mg of intramuscular of lorazepam, which only served to worsen Agatha's condition. The sign-out to the clinician who saw Agatha was that she was "psychotic" and likely needed to be transferred to an inpatient psychiatric unit.

We went into Agatha's room. She was petite, well-nourished, and generally healthy. She was inattentive, distractible, disorganized, and irritable, yelling about her husband and randomly reaching out into the air. She was able to state her name and birthdate, but was unable to correctly provide the current date, year, or day of the week. She did correctly identify the month. When asked about her present location, she responded that she was "in a church."

Darrell, who provided the aforementioned background information, was distraught and said that he was upset that he had heard a doctor, who never actually met with her, refer to her as "psychotic" based upon perfunctory details. After our assessment, we ordered a routine set of blood and urine laboratories, discontinued the benzodiazepines, and ordered a one-time dose of 5mg of olanzapine. We also performed a spot urinalysis and noticed positive leukocyte esterase and nitrites, as well as small amounts of protein and red blood cells. Suspecting a urinary tract infection, we ordered a dose of piperacillin/tazobactam.

No sooner had we written the orders for Agatha that we were told about, or heard, our next patient. According to the nurse, the patient was a young, 20-year-old male who was found running barefoot through the streets of Manhattan, shouting to passersby about the coming of the "Messiah" and the forthcoming apocalypse. A bystander called 911. When police and an ambulance arrived, the patient was found to be extremely agitated, belligerent, and uncooperative, saying the police were agents of the Devil. When he fled, yelling and screaming, the police called for backup. When they eventually caught up to the patient he attempted to fight them off with a twig. As per the report, it took five officers to apprehend the patient. He was placed in manual restraints for transportation on a gurney to a local emergency room.

The patient was brought into the emergency room during the previous shift on a gurney, with his arms and legs in restraints. He was screaming about the apocalypse and that the staff in the emergency room had to free him of his restraints in order to allow him to spread the word. Before his shift ended, our colleague in the emergency room ordered 5mg haloperidol, 2mg lorazepam, and 1mg of benztropine, all to be delivered intramuscularly, with an order to remove the patient from restraints if he were able to calm down and stop yelling.

Immediately after the patient's restraints were released he lunged at one of the male nurses and tackled him to the ground. He then got up and ran toward the exit screaming, "We are all going to die!" We, along with four security guards, raced to the entrance of the emergency room. Each one of us took one limb, and one person stabilized the head, and we took the person down. Although not an especially large person, the patient was inordinately strong. The four football lineman-sized security guards and we were only barely able to take down the patient and keep him down long enough for the nurse to inject 50mg of chlorpromazine into his buttocks. We then transferred him to a gurney and placed him back in manual restraints.

As we were walking back to the nurse's station to write our note about the agitated patient, a young woman entered the emergency room, speaking through barely comprehensible sobs about her daughter. She was distraught and walking so quickly and intently that she almost ran into two staff members, who, not understanding the situation, asked her to sit down and take a few deep breaths. She was given some water and a clinician was asked to speak with her. She explained that she had just put her infant daughter down for a nap and gone into her kitchen to prepare supper when she heard a choking sound coming from the child's crib. Discovering that the baby was not breathing and was turning cyanotic, the woman unsuccessfully tried to induce breathing before racing to the ER.

We asked where the child was at the moment. She explained that she, as a previous basic life support (BLS) instructor, had an infant bag valve mask at home. She had asked her 5-year-old son to remain with the infant in the car, delivering rescue breaths every two seconds to maximize oxygenation while the mother collected help from the emergency room. Upon hearing this we ran with the mother to her car, recruiting the help of the pediatric emergency room physician on the way. We found the son delivering rescue breaths to the infant who was strapped into a car seat, inexplicably covered with a sheet. Due to what appeared to be haste, the mother had locked her car keys in the car. Not being able to communicate with the young son through the windows, the backend of a tuning fork was used to gain entry through the passenger seat window and unlock the car. We grabbed the bag from the son and continued rescue breaths. The pediatric emergency room physician uncovered the infant.

Despite having seen thousands of patients in the ER and elsewhere, and hearing some of the most bizarre and incredible stories, the staff were not prepared for what transpired. Instead of finding an infant girl in the car seat, they found a toy doll of a young girl. It took a few moments to process what was happening and realize that there was no medical emergency. After confirming with the son, who was now frightened and crying loudly, that he had no sister and that his mother had asked him to provide rescue breaths to the doll, the clinician attempted to clarify the situation. Unfortunately, she was still very distraught, screaming about saving her daughter. She picked up the bag valve mask, placed it back on the doll's mouth and began providing rescue breaths. She kept pleading with us to save her daughter.

We brought the patient and her son into the ER and placed them in a closed room. The mother was given a small dose of oral olanzapine, after which she became calmer. A full medical work-up was conducted on the mother and no medical issues were found. The patient denied any psychiatric problems and held firmly to her belief that the doll was her daughter. In the meantime, her son was assessed for possible abuse or neglect. The social work team was consulted, making inquiries with child protective services. It emerged that she had a history of paranoid schizophrenia. While she had long been considered odd and suspicious at baseline, she met full criteria for the condition about two years prior, shortly after the sudden death of her husband in a road accident. Shocked and overwhelmed, the patient, who was several months pregnant with their second child – a daughter, miscarried. Since then, the patient had been hospitalized twice for psychotic episodes. In both instances, child protective services became involved, ensuring the son's care in her absences. Her brother looked after the boy as she underwent treatment.

While the content of the woman's delusion was stunning, this case, more importantly, highlights the importance of the social work team in an emergency setting and the need to always keep in mind minor children of impaired patients who are seen in an ER. It is critical to always ask patients who seem incapacitated whether or not they have any minor children and who is overseeing their care.

We went to check in on the young male who had been extremely agitated and was in restraints about two hours after he came into the emergency room. In the meantime, his urine toxicology came back positive for methamphetamine. Given that he had received a second round of intramuscular medications and was in restraints, we went to evaluate him for potential removal of the restraints. We went into the room accompanied by four security guards, which is called a "show of strength." The patient was lying on the gurney, calm, alert, and awake. He was fully oriented. He reported, in a much more calm and controlled way, that God was actively telling him that the world was coming to an end and that he had to spread the message to others. He made another reference to being John the Baptist. He was concerned that the clinician might be the Devil, pointing out the clinician's authoritative air, but also his facial hair, which was reminiscent of a drawing he once saw of a bearded Lucifer. He used profanity and said that he was convinced at that moment that there was no escape except to kill himself.

Although the patient was still acutely psychotic, endorsed suicidal ideation, and clearly required inpatient treatment, the clinician wrote an order for the restraints to be removed. While the man was hostile and delusional, he was no longer agitated. A security guard stood at the door of his room at all times for safety purposes. The authority to restrain a patient is a great responsibility and one that must be used judiciously. In general terms, manual restraints are used only when they are absolutely necessary and must be removed at the first opportunity.

There are two other important points about this case. First, this patient, who had no history of psychosis, was floridly psychotic, likely precipitated by abuse and overuse of methamphetamine. Drug-induced psychosis can be quite severe and, in certain individuals so predisposed, occur after even one dose of a substance, depending on the size of the dose. Here, the patient had been using methamphetamine for several days. Drug-induced psychosis can be every bit or even more severe than psychosis not involving an illicit drug and often manifests as acute episodes involving severe delusions, hallucinations, and agitation. Individuals with drug-induced psychosis can be particularly difficult to manage, not only because of the severity of their symptoms, but also because they become inordinately strong, almost in a superhuman way. It is very common for people experiencing a drug-induced psychosis to lose their inhibitions and develop such strength, as exhibited when this patient required several large guards to hold him down so that injectable medications could be administered.

Second, while antipsychotic medications are used on a daily basis to treat psychotic symptoms and to prevent relapse, they are also often the best medication choice for acute agitation in the context of severe psychosis, as displayed by this patient. Antipsychotic medications, especially when paired with benzodiazepines such as lorazepam, can be highly effective (1). Perhaps the most often used and effective combination is the "five, two and one" trio of 5mg of haloperidol, 2mg of lorazepam and 1mg of benztropine (to prevent extrapyramidal side effects from haloperidol). In this case, this regimen was only mildly effective, so the clinician tried another common medication, intramuscular chlorpromazine, which is also quite effective. Other medications that are commonly used for acute agitation and psychosis in an emergency room are intramuscular ziprasidone, olanzapine, aripiprazole, and benzodiazepines alone.

Our next few patients were typical of patients in the emergency room. We had two more cases of people with severe agitation secondary to drug-induced psychoses. We also had a third patient, "Arthur," with drug-induced psychosis, brought in from home. In the context of using cocaine for three straight days, he stopped sleeping and grew paranoid about his neighbors. Earlier in the day he was found with a baseball bat trying to break into the house next door, which was, fortunately, unoccupied at the time. When Arthur's wife saw what he was doing, she called 911 and he was brought to the ER. Upon arrival he was delusional but calm. He explained that the reason that he had approached his neighbor's house was that he was "tired of how loud they are at night." He reported that their voices and yelling routinely prevented him from obtaining a full night's rest. Arthur denied wanting to harm anyone, claiming to have brought a baseball bat with him when approaching the neighbors' home because he was unsure that they would otherwise hear him knocking on their door. Arthur's wife reported that there was actually no noise from the people next door at night or at any time. It appeared, therefore, that Arthur was experiencing auditory hallucinations. He was kept in the emergency room for 24 hours and given low doses of risperidone. During his stay, he slept for 16 hours and received a total of 2mg of risperidone. By the end of his observation period, his delusions had almost completely resolved. He reported feeling much better and that he understood the effect of cocaine on his life. His wife related that he had abused the drug in the past and recently "fallen off of the wagon." She stated that his current mental status was his baseline. Arthur committed to engaging in an outpatient substance abuse therapy and was subsequently discharged.

Another patient, "Ashley," visited the emergency room, reporting concern about her pregnancy of the past six months; specifically, that she had not felt any kicking throughout the day. She appeared four to five months pregnant and was taken to the obstetrics room in the ER. Upon ultrasound, however, the physicians were unable to locate a pregnancy. This was confirmed by a serum pregnancy test, which indicated that the patient was, in fact, not pregnant. Psychiatry was consulted. The patient turned out to be very well known to the colleague who now evaluated her, having encountered her many times in another local emergency room. The patient had a chronic delusion that she was pregnant and went to an ER approximately twice a year with the same complaint that her baby had stopped moving or kicking. The delusion returned whenever the patient stopped her antipsychotic medications. Otherwise, the patient functioned well, held a full-time job, and was married. With the patient's consent and request, the clinician spoke with her outpatient psychiatrist, confirmed her history, restarted her risperidone, and discharged her back to her home with her husband. She agreed to see her own psychiatrist the following day.

The next patient was "Liam," a 45-year-old male with a history of schizophrenia and head trauma following a severe motor vehicle accident. He was sent from his adult group home for bizarre behavior. Although impaired from his chronic, treatment-refractory schizophrenia and comorbid traumatic brain injury, he was generally able to manage independently in this setting. The staff at the group home would supply his daily medications. The group home reported that they had sent Liam to the ER following several days of diminished hygiene, defecation on the floors, and repeatedly exposing himself to other patients. We were also told that he was eating his own feces, the clinical term for which is coprophagia.

We met with Liam. He was very pleasant, childlike, and highly disinhibited, the latter being typical for some patients who have suffered traumatic brain injuries. Liam explained that he had been exposing himself to other people in the group home because he "thought they would like that." When asked about why he was eating feces, he replied that he was experiencing constipation and would insert one finger into his anus in order to encourage evacuation of rectum. After doing so, he would taste his feces to make sure there were no toxins in his system.

We performed several tests on Liam to try to understand what might have been responsible for his decompensation, including an MRI and blood and urine tests. We also obtained blood levels of his clozapine, which were extremely low, indicating that he had not been taking his medications. The psychiatrist asked Liam about this. The patient reported that he did not like how his medications made him feel, so would put them in his mouth and keep them in his cheek until he went back to his room, then would spit them into the toilet. The case emphasizes that potential nonadherence with medications must always be considered when a patient with schizophrenia presents with a sudden relapse.

After finishing with the last patient, we sat down at the very end of the emergency room and took a quick break to grab an energy bar from the snack machine. While eating the bar, we noticed a young woman sitting on a gurney arching her back in a rhythmic motion, as if she were trying to very gradually lean further and further back, with a deep arch in her back. Her left forearm was overpronating and her right arm was supinating. She seemed to be trying to speak, but instead was only crying. It emerged that the woman was a cancer patient who had come in an hour earlier complaining of muscle stiffness. Upon examination, the attending physician was unable to find anything wrong with the patient, prompting him to conclude that her symptoms were "all in her head." He prescribed 600mg of ibuprofen and planned to discharge her with the instruction to follow-up with her treating oncologist.

We went over to the patient and inquired how she was feeling and why she had come into the emergency room. At this point, she was almost completely leaning back and was unable to articulate any words. In addition, her eyes began to deviate upwards, moving further and further up in their sockets. Immediately upon seeing this, we ordered 50mg of intramuscular diphenhydramine from the nurse and administered it into the patient's arm. We waited by her side, providing support and encouragement, while waiting for the medication to work. Within 30 seconds, the patient's movements and rigidity began to subside and she assumed a more normal posture. About three minutes later, the woman's movements had completely resolved. The patient, whom we will call "Matilda," was quite relieved, wiping tears from her eyes and asking what, exactly, had happened to her. We asked her if she had taken any medications that day, such as metoclopramide, prochlorperazine, or any psychiatric medications. She reported that she had developed intractable nausea from her chemotherapy and was prescribed trifluoperazine by her oncologist. She took her first dose three hours before heading to the ER. She developed stiffness, severe pain, difficulty speaking, and generally "did not feel right." She was concerned that the physicians in the emergency room did not understand what was happening to her. She said that she thought that she was going to die. She was instructed to keep a 50mg pill of diphenhydramine with her for the rest of the day and speak with her oncologist about a medication besides trifluoperazine.

Matilda had, in fact, suffered from an oculogyric crisis, a severe form of dystonia. Dystonia is the most acute of the extrapyramidal side effects associated with antipsychotic medications. It occurs on a timescale of minutes to days. It is associated with the so-called first-generation antipsychotic medications, such as haloperidol, trifluoperazine, and fluphenazine, as well as related antiemetic medications, including metoclopramide and prochlorperazine. It is most associated with first-generation antipsychotic medications, and especially those with the highest potency (i.e., those that require the lowest doses to be effective such as haloperidol and trifluoperazine, whereas the risk is lower with medications such as chlorpromazine or thioridazine). It typically involves involuntary, sustained muscular contractions of the face, extremities, neck, torso, or larynx. Rarely, laryngeal dystonia can be deadly. Acute dystonic reactions usually occur when a person first starts a medication or after he or she increases the dose. These reactions can be painful and, when someone has such a reaction, the individual often refuses to take the same offending medication again. Treatment with anticholinergic medications or benzodiazepines can be effective, either acutely or prophylactically.

It was five minutes before the end of our shift. We were tired, drained, and wanted to go home. But before doing so, we checked in on Agatha. She was propped up in her bed, eating breakfast. Darrell, who had stayed all night in the emergency room, was sitting in a chair alongside her. Agatha reported that she was tired, but felt significantly better. She was fully oriented and more attentive upon interview. She admitted to not totally remembering what had happened over the previous 24 hours. We told Agatha and her husband that it looked like she had been delirious, probably precipitated by the combination of a urinary tract infection and benzodiazepines.

Delirium is a common cause of psychotic symptoms, especially in older individuals. By definition, delirium always has a medical cause. Consequently, the treatment is always symptomatic, in addition to being aimed at the goal of identifying and treating the root cause. Delirium is more common in the medically infirm. Common causes are medications, such as benzodiazepines and anticholinergics, especially in the elderly; drug withdrawal; or medical conditions, such as infections, procedures that include anesthesia, marked insomnia, metabolic or chemical imbalances, or terminal illness. After identifying and treating the underlying cause or causes, other treatments might include antipsychotic medications, frequent orientation, reassurance, and maintenance of a normal sleep-wake cycle.

Agatha presented with a standard case of delirium, which, unfortunately, was incorrectly conceptualized when she first arrived in the ER. After we explained the situation to the patient and her husband, Agatha was advised to remain one more night on an inpatient medical unit for observation and a proper tapering of her lorazepam.

As we walked out of the emergency room, we could not help but smile, very happy that we were able to make a difference in Agatha and Darrell's lives, eager for our next shift.

Reference

1. Buchanan RW, Kreyenbuhl J, Kelly DL, Noel JM, Boggs DL, Fischer BA, Himelhoch S, Fang B, Peterson E, Aquino PR, Keller W. The 2009 schizophrenia PORT psychopharmacological treatment recommendations and summary statements. *Schizophr Bull.* 2009;36(1):71–93.

7

IMPAIRED FUNCTIONING AND DOWNWARD SHIFT IN FUNCTIONING IN SCHIZOPHRENIA

One of the saddest patients we have come across during our years in psychiatry was "Reggie." He came from a family that had substantial amounts of money and New England pedigree. They owned property all over the Eastern seaboard and French Riviera. Family members tended to receive their education at Ivy League schools and work at top firms in New York City.

However, their family history of psychiatric illness, and in particular psychotic illness, ran as deep as their pockets and pedigree. The first known record of psychiatric illness in their family came from the Civil War era. One of their great-great-great-great grandfathers was discharged from the Union Army because of a delusion that, at night, the animals in the forests would anthropomorphize and come together for drinks, tea, and coffee. Other officers would find the ancestor trying to interact and speak with forest animals at night. One time he crept up on an unsuspecting deer which charged at him and punctured his leg. Other family members have become severely psychotic and lived their lives as hermits in the hills of West Virginia, often found eating out of pig troughs on farms. More recent family members have populated the wards of long-term psychiatric hospitals in Massachusetts, Maryland, and Texas, among others.

Reggie first came to our attention after responding to an advertisement for a clinical research study using Magnetic Resonance Imaging, or MRI, to look at the brains of people with psychosis. MRI has been used in psychiatric research for approximately 30 years now, and has revealed several very important findings, including that people with schizophrenia have larger ventricles (the fluid filled spaces of the brain) than other people (1), as well as smaller hippocampi (2), which are the regions responsible for short-term memory. Most importantly, MRI has proved once and for all that schizophrenia is a "brain disorder," rather than a purely "functional" disorder outside of the realm of traditional medicine.

Reggie was a tall, relatively athletic appearing man in his late 20s, severely disheveled and unkempt. His clothes were dirty and tattered, he was malodorous and had long hair and a grown-out beard that appeared to have not been groomed in years. He was pleasant and cooperative. Perhaps most striking, and unexpected, about Reggie was his accent and demeanor. Though he had spent essentially his whole life in New England, and particularly New York City, he spoke and acted as if he were from Australia, using words such as "crikey" and "ripper." He also insisted on bringing gifts to every visit, which usually consisted of old newspapers and shoelaces that he had found on the street.

Reggie had grown up in the lap of luxury. He had attended the best private elementary and high schools. He was a successful athlete, having played basketball and tennis, and run track in high school. He graduated high school at the top of his class and went to a prominent college. At the time of his graduation from high school, he was in a serious relationship with the daughter of a national politician from New York.

However, it was in his first year of college when Reggie developed schizophrenia. He began to isolate and skip class. He stopped spending time with his girlfriend and stopped playing sports. He became very interested with the occult and supernatural phenomena. He spent most of his time reading about these subject areas. He stopped shaving and showering. Eventually, his roommate complained to their dormitory resident adviser about the patient's behavior. The patient's parents, who were extremely supportive, caring, and knowledgeable about mental illness, took Reggie to see the family's psychiatrist, who began the patient on 1mg twice daily of risperidone.

Reggie took the rest of the semester off to recover and began an intensive outpatient program. An intensive outpatient program is exactly how it sounds. Patients go to this type of program as outpatients, usually three to five days a week, and engage in groups, vocational training, and individual treatment. He made a near full recovery and was able to return to college the next semester.

Reggie did not, however, last very long in college. Immediately after returning to college, and without his parents' encouragement to take his medications, he stopped taking them. He quickly relapsed and had to leave college again. This time, however, Reggie refused to restart any medications. He was very delusional and not attending to his own hygiene, but refused to take any medications. In addition, there were no grounds for the family to force medication against the patient's will. No one was able to convince Reggie to take medications. Over the years, Reggie's condition worsened, although not necessarily directly due to his psychotic symptoms. He became less interested in living with his parents and began spending time on the streets. He eventually spent all his time on the streets and was homeless. At first, his family would visit him, bring him food and clothing, and try to convince him to come back with them, but he refused. Reggie was very happy and content living on the streets. He would spend every day at the public library, reading about the occult and supernatural phenomena. He was certain an alien race was "among us" and was using laser beams to try to steal his thoughts and control his mind. Reggie began wearing a baseball cap lined, on the inside, with aluminum foil to prevent laser beams from penetrating his brain.

Shortly before presenting to our clinic, Reggie developed the idea to invent a device that would produce clones of himself that would confuse the aliens into thinking that they were the real Reggie, rather than him. However, in order to obtain such a device, Reggie would need money, and he had no interest in asking his family for money. Therefore, Reggie responded to our advertisement for a research study.

During our initial interview, Reggie explained to us his concerns about aliens and that they were using laser beams to try to steal his thoughts. He showed us his aluminum foil-lined baseball hat and explained to us how it worked. He went on to describe a number of other symptoms, including that he had always felt "different ... like in another dimension than everyone else in the world, kind of like I am living in the same world as other people but they cannot notice me." When asked if Reggie was dead, he said that he does not believe he is dead, "or else why would the aliens want to steal my thoughts." He explained that he used to experience thought broadcasting, in which his thoughts would be broadcast aloud to anyone willing to listen, but that lining his baseball cap with aluminum foil also solved this problem. Reggie reported that, about once a week, his dreams would come true, which he described as having some control of nature, like a demigod – "why else would the aliens be so interested in my thoughts? They want to unlock the powers of my brain." We asked Reggie if he had ever seen the aliens. He had not, but reported that he could "sense" them and suspected that they were advanced beings,

> not like the silly depictions of aliens in the movies and on television, but more sophisticated, abstract, godlike, and metaphysical. The rules of nature do not apply to them. They view me as the highest form of life next to them and are intrigued by how I could have evolved so quickly and from such a primitive race.

Reggie was not overtly paranoid about people, but did explain that,

> if anyone were to find out about who I am and how powerful I am, they would probably not leave me alone. I don't think that these people are bad, just jealous, primitive, and simple-minded. But I do have to be careful. I have not told anyone about my powers or what I know about aliens in years. This is partly because I don't want to be treated differently, but also because it is possible that they might be controlled by the aliens themselves, so I am generally mindful about with whom I speak. Yesterday I was in a convenience store buying a soft drink. I was waiting in line behind a man who was carrying his baby. The baby was looking directly at me. He was

very odd looking and would not stop looking at me. I suspected that he was under the control of the aliens. Fortunately, I had just forgotten to replace my hat on my head after using the restroom. The baby stopped looking at me when I replaced my hat.

Reggie denied a belief in God or any omnipotent being, besides himself and the aliens who "simply evolved" to become more sophisticated and complex life forms. He reported that he did, several times a week, hear transmissions, like radio transmissions, with moderate amounts of static. He did not hear voices, but suspected that what he heard were alien transmissions. He reported that these were not bothersome to him, but rather that he was happy to have them in order to stay updated on their plans and movements.

While Reggie was sometimes linear and goal-directed, he was more often tangential and circumstantial; overly abstract; loose; vague; and idiosyncratic. He was hyperloquacious at times. In some instances he noticed his own disorganization and restructured himself; however, there were numerous points at which he needed prompts and questions to be reoriented. He was responsive to this structuring.

We engaged Reggie in our research. He declined clinical treatment per se, though often asked to meet with us to discuss his life and ideas. We regularly encouraged Reggie to take medications and engage in therapy, though he always declined. After several months of engagement in our clinic, Reggie revealed why he decided to never take medications. First, Reggie's insight was only partial. He understood that he had schizophrenia and unusual ideas, but denied that he needed any treatment for it. He reported that risperidone helped him to sleep and think more clearly, but also that it caused side effects that he did not like at all and so decided he would never take medications again. In particular, Reggie reported that, while taking risperidone, he noticed that he had developed small amounts of breast tissue and, at one point, noticed minor galactorrhea. He also reported that he had no libido while taking risperidone and had erectile dysfunction. He reported that he was so embarrassed by these side effects that he had actually stopped taking his medications well before he went back to school. We educated Reggie about the side effects of risperidone. We confirmed that, in some people, schizophrenia medications, and especially risperidone, can increase a hormone called prolactin which can lead to gynecomastia, galactorrhea, and sexual dysfunction. We explained that Reggie could take another medication that is much less likely to case galactorrhea, such as a second-generation antipsychotic medication like aripiprazole or quetiapine. Reggie refused and said he would never take a psychiatric medication again.

Importantly, despite Reggie's susbstantial positive symptoms and moderate disorganization, he had few negative symptoms. This was important for many reasons, including that Reggie was very interested in developing a relationship with a woman. This added greater significance to why Reggie was so resistant to medications after having experienced sexual dysfunction with risperidone. Further, this added to Reggie's overall sense of low self-worth. He explained that he had a poor sense of himself from a very young age. Even though he was considered to be athletic and social, he reported that he never felt comfortable around women. He went on to say that his father was a stereotypically masculine, "alpha" male who, even when married, frequently had relationships with many women. Reggie was very traumatized by how his father acted, both because of how badly his mother felt about his father's relationships, but also because he felt that his father was very critical of him for not being as aggressive, cocky, and stereotypically masculine. Reggie's father frequently encouraged his sons (Reggie had an older brother named Robert), from their teenage years, to have relationships with as many women as possible. At family outings, he would point out young women whom they should meet. Even when Reggie was seeing his girlfriend his father would suggest that he meet other women in order to "keep from getting bored." Reggie thought this behavior was disgusting. Reggie loved his father and appreciated his support throughout his life, but wanted to be a completely different person than his father.

Over time, we began to understand that Reggie benefitted greatly from coming to see us. Although he only, ostensibly, came to us for research, he greatly appreciated the support, attention, respect, and feedback that we would give him. It also appeared that Reggie began to develop a strong transference to us, to the point that he began to view us as father figures. He developed an obvious desire to gain our acceptance and approval. An example of this is how hard he would try to make us laugh. It got to the point that his research sessions with us would turn into performances. He would spend whole sessions describing his life by joking about himself, as a self-deprecating stand-up comedian might.

Despite Reggie's strong alliance with us, and our persistent attempts to convince him to try medications and engage in treatment, he adamantly refused medications. He continued to prefer being homeless and living on the streets to taking medications and living with his family. At this point, he had been living on the streets for several years. His family had tried endlessly to help him, but he refused. Once they found out that Reggie was receiving care in our clinic, they reached out to us and asked us to help them convince Reggie to go back to living with them, or at least allow them to put him up in some sort of shelter, but he would always and adamantly refuse. In fact, despite his otherwise pleasant, somewhat emotional demeanor, any discussion about or mention of his family would send Reggie into a very dark and isolated mindset.

Reggie refused to discuss his family at all, but, as far as we could tell, Reggie was not overtly paranoid about his family, nor were any of his psychotic symptoms necessarily related to his family. He simply refused to have them as part of his life in any way, preferring to live a life of poverty, hunger, and simplicity. He had no money and refused to live in the shelter system. Several times a month he would come to the clinic and describe instances in which he was beaten up on the streets or propositioned in other ways. He would occasionally ask to participate in a research study, such as an MRI study, when he needed some money, but otherwise was just happy with his current state.

Transience, or living in a lower social class, is not uncommon in schizophrenia. Much of it likely has to do with the effects of the illness on attention, memory, planning, sociality, and demeanor (i.e., negative symptoms, cognitive deficits, disorganization) which make it harder to work, make money, and stay out of poverty – i.e., these patients experience a downward social mobility on account of their condition (3). Those patients with social and family networks that can support them tend to do better and are usually able to stay off the streets. Fortunately, this is relatively common and prevents many individuals from unavoidable homelessness and poverty, which themselves worsen schizophrenia and produce a cycle of homelessness, hospitalization, and poverty from which it is hard to remove oneself.

The decision to live in severe poverty seemed to be unrelated to Reggie's psychotic symptoms. We have seen this in our careers, but only a handful of times, and such situations are usually related to a specific delusion or hallucination that would make the decision logical, though psychotic. It is not clear what this represented for Reggie. It is possible that his choice to live in severe poverty was more generally related to the disorganization and feelings of being emotionally overwhelmed in a more structured, abundant society.

Consistent with Reggie's otherwise surprising and counter-logical way of life was his refusal to accept treatment with medications. While we could not be certain that treatment with antipsychotic medications would have had any beneficial effect on Reggie's symptoms, the odds would have been in his favor. Especially early in one's illness, for example in the first several years, medications can be effective in upwards of 80% of patients in terms of substantially reducing symptoms (4). Their effectiveness decreases the longer a person has symptoms, but usually remains to some degree for most people (5, 6). However, Reggie would always refuse medications and managed to stay out of hospitals, jails, and other settings in which he could have been required to take medications. Reggie's case was particularly unfortunate because he was a known responder to medications. Therefore, the chances that he would have responded to medications was extremely high. Of course, we described this to Reggie as well, though he continued to refuse to take medications. As of the writing of this book, Reggie had schizophrenia for ten years and had never taken any medications after he first tried risperidone. He continued to live on the streets in severe poverty, often hungry and beaten, coming on time to the clinic for his weekly therapy sessions.

References

1. Degreef G, Ashtari M, Bogerts B, Bilder RM, Jody DN, Alvir JM, Lieberman JA. Volumes of ventricular system subdivisions measured from magnetic resonance images in first-episode schizophrenic patients. *Arch Gen Psychiatry*. 1992;49(7):531–537.

2. Bogerts B, Lieberman JA, Ashtari M, Bilder RM, Degreef G, Lerner G, Johns C, Masiar S. Hippocampus-amygdala volumes and psychopathology in chronic schizophrenia. *Biol Psychiatry*. 1993;33(4):236–246.
3. Bromet EJ, Fennig S. Epidemiology and natural history of schizophrenia. *Biol Psychiatry*. 1999;46(7):871–881.
4. Robinson DG, Woerner MG, Alvir JM, Geisler S, Koreen A, Sheitman B, Chakos M, Mayerhoff D, Bilder R, Goldman R, Lieberman JA. Predictors of treatment response from a first episode of schizophrenia or schizoaffective disorder. *Am J Psychiatry*. 1999;156(4):544–549.
5. Sheitman BB, Lieberman JA. The natural history and pathophysiology of treatment resistant schizophrenia. *J Psychiatr Res*. 1998;32(3–4):143–150.
6. Lieberman JA, Sheitman B, Chakos M, Robinson D, Schooler N, Keith S. The development of treatment resistance in patients with schizophrenia: a clinical and pathophysiologic perspective. *J Clin Psychopharmacol*. 1998;18(2 Suppl 1):20S–24S.

8
FIXED-FALSE BELIEFS

"Joy" started her morning as she always does, waking up at 7:00am and checking online news financial websites to keep updated on all the latest in technology and business. This morning she was very pleased to catch a short feature about herself on one of the popular science and technology morning news shows that was profiling the most important people in the field of technology under the age of 40. She felt that they had portrayed her story well; that she left college after several years in order to put all of her time, effort, and money into her invention of a non-invasive way to measure blood sugar in people with diabetes using infrared technology; that this invention would not only be worth billions of dollars but would reshape diagnostics in medicine; and that this invention would catapult Joy's name into discussions of leading thinkers, entrepreneurs, and inventors. Joy was extremely excited about her invention and the interest she had received and was patiently waiting for a letter in the mail from the United States Patent and Notification Office indicating that her patent was approved, which would be the last step before receiving "money, success, and admiration." However, most important to Joy was that her idea would make it so much easier for people with diabetes, such as her mother Angela, to monitor their blood sugar without painful pin pricks.

Joy loved her mother and had an unusually close bond with her. Joy's father left the family when Joy was very young, shortly after they immigrated from Western Africa to the United States. Joy's mother worked several jobs to provide for her. Joy had always felt that her mother sacrificed a great deal, including her own health and happiness, in order to give her a better life. Her mother never dated or married after her father left them. Working so many hours left Joy's mother very little time to focus on her own health. Over the years she gained substantial amounts of weight and eventually developed diabetes. Joy had always felt a desire to pay her mother back for sacrificing so much for Joy. Joy's invention would provide more than enough financial support to allow her mother to quit her jobs and have an opportunity to relax and enjoy her life after decades of working multiple, low paying jobs.

Joy described herself as always having enjoyed social interactions, but constantly feeling that she was smarter and destined for something greater than her friends. She reported that her friends were "generally ok and good people," but that they simply did not have her "intellect, ambition, or ingenuity." She had three good friends growing up, whom she had not seen in over a decade. She spent most of her free time at home with her mother. She had never been married and had no children. She had one relatively serious romantic relationship as a 19-year-old, lasting four months. She remained attracted to people, but stated that she felt her relationship prospects were hampered because "there are few guys out there who are comfortable with being with a woman smarter than they are and who will have more money than they will."

Joy had never been in special education. She had never been left back in school. She had been in standard classes in middle school and high school and described herself as generally a "B+" student across her lifetime. She explained that she did not perform better because she was "never interested in the material covered in class" and felt that "it was a waste of my time and talent."

Joy's symptoms began when she was 16 years old. As described above, Joy began to have thoughts that she was destined for great things and would become a billionaire. She began explaining this to her teachers and friends. She also began to think that a famous actor was secretly in love with her and that he would signal his love for her in his movies and during television interviews. She would also occasionally hear the actor's voice saying "I love you" even when nobody was around, which she would interpret as further proof of their connection, i.e., that they were able to communicate even when not in each other's presence (of note, Joy had never actually met the actor in person nor communicated with him in any way).

Joy had a number of other symptoms during the first few years of her illness, particularly when she first became ill, and also during relapses. Namely, she would at times describe a sense of nihilism – that the world was coming to an end and life was meaningless. She would not be able to explain how or why this was the case, but would describe the world as "vanity" and question "what the point of anything is anymore." During one of her more significant relapses she reported that she had lost the use of her legs. For this, Joy required one week on an inpatient medical unit. Because of how dramatic and complete Joy's paralysis was, her physician wanted to do a full workup to confirm that they were not missing a medical cause of her condition. After a week of extensive medical testing, the team of physicians decided that Joy's paralysis was mostly likely related to her schizophrenia and she was admitted to an inpatient psychiatric unit for two weeks where the dose of her antipsychotic medication was increased. On the tenth day that Joy was on the unit, she woke up with full use of her legs and went on as if her paralysis had never happened.

During another of Joy's relapses, at a time when she had run out of medications and had not told her mother or psychiatrist, Joy began to develop the feeling that people in the streets were able to hear her thoughts and insert thoughts into her mind. Joy became very upset by this. One day when Joy went to the grocery store to buy milk and eggs, she thought that an elderly lady who was shopping next to her could hear her thoughts, which were being broadcast aloud for anyone to hear. She also thought that this elderly lady was trying to place the thought in Joy's mind to grab a child who was playing nearby with her mother. Panicked, Joy dropped her groceries and ran out of the store. Thereafter, she refused to leave her home for 14 days straight due to the fear of being around people when they were able to do these things. Eventually Joy's mother called her psychiatrist who sent in a refill of Joy's medication. Joy's mother picked the medication up from the pharmacy for Joy to restart them. Within several days, Joy's symptoms improved so that she was able to go out in public again.

These symptoms began to cause problems at school, though Joy was able to begin treatment relatively quickly, thanks to her school counselor who referred Joy to a psychiatrist. She was able to complete high school after which she enrolled in a local community college, taking approximately one class a semester, as well as working part-time. Joy first began working at age 18 as staff at a bowling alley and then worked as a waitress at age 19. She did not excel at either and was let go from her position as a waitress for ignoring tables and occasionally stealing other waitresses' tips. When asked why she would steal other waitresses' tips she responded that she needed the money to invest in her latest invention. She also sometimes worked as a nanny for pay. Joy occasionally worked temporary jobs, such as working in tax preparation or temporary administrative work. She reported using small amount of cannabis and alcohol in her lifetime, no more than five times each, mostly while in high school.

Joy's condition waxed and waned for many years. Her feelings of superiority and grandiosity generally never totally remitted regardless of how Joy's other symptoms responded to treatment, though were more substantial at times, while her hallucinations and other delusions tended to remit with treatment. She initially tried haloperidol and chlorpromazine, followed by risperidone and ziprasidone. She eventually settled on 300mg of quetiapine.

Joy clearly met criteria for schizophrenia based on her many months to years of delusions and hallucinations. In particular, Joy's condition was dominated by her many delusions. Delusions are beliefs that are definitively not true but about which a person has complete conviction. They may be bizarre (e.g., being controlled by aliens) or plausible (e.g., being monitored by the FBI) but must be untrue, by definition. Delusions are distinct from hallucinations. Delusions are thoughts that are unreal though believed to be true. Hallucinations are actual perceptions or sensations related to sight, touch, hearing, smell, or taste that are unreal but experienced by an individual; for example, smelling something when there is nothing to smell. Often, especially in schizophrenia, the themes of the hallucinations and delusions may be related. For example, someone may have auditory hallucinations of voices telling her that the FBI is monitoring oneself and also believe that one is being monitored by hidden cameras. Another example would be that one hears God talking to oneself and believes oneself to be a messenger of God.

Delusions are among the most common symptoms in schizophrenia and are one of the five main symptoms of schizophrenia, along with hallucinations, disorganized speech, disorganized behavior, and negative symptoms (to meet criteria for schizophrenia, patients must meet at least two of these criteria [one must be delusions, hallucinations, or disorganized speech] for one month with some signs of the disorder for at least six months, unless they receive treatment). There are many different types of delusions. One type of delusion is the persecutory delusion. In this type of delusion, one believes that they are being worked against, targeted, or unfairly treated in some way. A person having persecutory delusions is often described as being "paranoid." This is perhaps the most common type of delusion experienced by individuals with schizophrenia, though it was not experienced by Joy. An example of a persecutory delusion would be thinking that one is being monitored by cameras that no one can see or that a government agency is planning to assassinate someone when that is not true.

Religious delusions are another very common type of delusion and involve religious ideas that are impossible, such as thinking that one is a deity or speaks directly with God. Religious delusions are distinct from religious overzealousness.

Grandiose delusions involve the idea that one is extremely powerful, important, rich, or valuable in some way. Joy's delusions about her idea for an invention and becoming a billionaire from it are examples of grandiose delusions. Other examples may include thinking that one is a king or leader of a country when that is not the case or when someone believes that they have a superior intellect when they do not, such as what Joy experienced.

Nihilistic delusions involve feeling like one's life is extremely empty and purposeless or that life is unreal. Joy would occasionally have thoughts such as these during relapses. Another type of delusion that is relatively common, and which Joy also experienced, is a delusion of reference. A delusion of reference is experienced when someone believes that remarks, objects, or events which are otherwise insignificant, or unrelated to them, have personal meaning or significance. Joy's feelings that events in an actor's movies were signs to her are examples of delusions of reference. Joy's feelings that the actor was in love with her is another type of delusion, referred to as an erotomanic delusion. Erotomanic delusions are the false belief that someone is in love with them. This often has a grandiose component, such as in Joy's case in which she believed that a famous movie star was in love with her.

Joy also experienced somatic delusions. Somatic delusions are false beliefs that have to do with physical or bodily functioning or a medical condition. Joy's experiences that her legs were not working is an example of a somatic delusion.

Delusions of mind reading are when somebody thinks that people can read their minds. These are distinct from delusions of thought broadcasting, endorsed by Joy, which are the belief that one's thoughts are being broadcast aloud, such as how Joy thought that the elderly lady at the grocery store could hear her thoughts because they were being broadcast aloud. Joy also experienced delusions of thought insertion. These are the belief that another person is literally placing thoughts into one's mind. In Joy's case, she thought that the elderly lady at the grocery store was trying to place thoughts into her mind to grab a child who was playing nearby with her mother. Delusions of thought withdrawal are the belief that people are able to remove thoughts from a person's mind. Delusions of being controlled involve the actual belief that another being, human or otherwise, has gained control of their thoughts and/or actions. Individuals with delusions of control feel that the only reason they are acting the way they are acting is because of the outside agent having commandeered their body and/or mind.

Delusions of jealousy and guilt are also relatively common delusions observed in individuals with schizophrenia. A delusion of jealousy often has to do with thinking that someone's partner or spouse is cheating on them. Delusions of guilt are when someone feels that they have committed a great and unforgivable act or sin. For example, someone might wrongly believe that they were responsible for an earthquake that killed many people, even though this is not possible.

As Joy was leaving her home, she told her mother she would be back in a few hours after running some errands. Her first errand was to go to the tailor and pick up her custom-made eyeglasses. Joy had invested $2000 in designer eyeglasses and jewelry. While Joy would normally never make such purchases, she realized that, with the imminent revelation and mainstream success of her invention would come numerous meetings and interviews with investors and journalists and she wanted to look the part. Joy knew that her mother would never allow her to spend $2000 on anything, let alone accessories, so Joy obtained a cash loan from a pawn shop. As collateral, Joy took her mother's family heirloom, a gold necklace with a golden cross brought over by her mother's ancestors when they immigrated to Western Africa from Eastern Africa in the 17th century, and gave it to the pawn shop.

Although it was a cloudy and rainy day, Joy began wearing her glasses and jewelry immediately after purchasing them. The glasses and jewelry made Joy look the way she felt — confident, intelligent, and unique. As she walked out of the store wearing the designer glasses and jewelry she saw many familiar faces and people from her neighborhood looking at her, as she was out of place wearing such expensive items in her relatively modest neighborhood. Joy liked the people in her neighborhood and the neighborhood itself, but always felt that she did not quite belong there and that she was destined for greater things. Joy felt very good about herself knowing that when she were to become rich from her invention she would give back to her community.

The next errand was for Joy to see her therapist. Joy felt very comfortable speaking with her therapist. Joy felt that her therapist was kind, available, and supportive. The therapist did not seem to understand the invention very well, but that would be expected as not many people would be able to understand how using infrared technology could produce blood sugar readings. Further, with Joy's impending financial success and fame, she felt that she would need to see a therapist, like most celebrities and important people.

Today's therapy session focused on how Joy would be able to handle such a drastic change in her life after her invention became patented and she began to receive investments in her ideas. Joy's therapist suggested that Joy try not to make too many changes to her life just yet, or too quickly, and to allow things to play out and settle before making any big decisions. Joy's therapist also complimented Joy on her new glasses and jewelry and asked her how she was able to afford them. Joy explained that she obtained a cash loan from a pawn shop, using her mother's necklace as collateral, but that this was irrelevant since before too long Joy would not only be able to buy back her mother's necklace, but also buy any amount of designer items and jewelry she would like. Joy also thought that it was unusual that her therapist recommended that she consider a medication reevaluation with a psychiatrist since she only had stress related to "real-life situations" rather than any sort of chemical imbalance. Joy told her therapist that the only reason she was on quetiapine was for "insomnia" and that she did not think that she needed any other medications. Joy was very appreciative that her therapist offered her very practical advice and would not allow her to get too far ahead of herself, but did feel that the therapist was, at times, slightly jealous of her. Namely, Joy was only in her early thirties, had dropped out of college, and invented one of the greatest medical breakthroughs of the last decade, while her therapist was twice her age, had a PhD, and was still making a modest living by seeing ten patients a day. Joy felt sympathetic toward her therapist that she was not able to make as much of her life as Joy was and was reminded about her feelings of appreciation that her therapist was pleasant and available and had been willing to treat Joy even before becoming rich and famous.

Joy left her therapy session with feelings of well-being and calm, eager to check the mailbox for the approval letter from the United States Patent and Notification Office. Joy did not find any such letter in her mailbox. She asked her mother if she had perhaps found the letter herself. She had not. Joy's mother asked Joy to tell her about her day. Joy spent almost two hours telling her mother about her day, including the news story profiling her invention, her therapy session, and her appreciation of her therapist, how she was going to help out people in the neighborhood after she became rich and famous, as well as how her mother was going to be able to quit her job and move into a large house with a pool and maids and servants so that she would never have to work again. Joy even told her about her glasses and jewelry and how happy and confident she felt when wearing them. Her mother smiled the whole time, telling Joy how wonderful her idea was and how professional she looked in her accessories.

After speaking with her mother, Joy prepared for bed. While doing so she was able to watch another profile about her on the television during a one-hour show on the future of chronic diseases, such as diabetes. Joy turned off the television thinking about what a great service she will be doing for mankind and fell asleep with thoughts of excitement about the next day, knowing that tomorrow could be the day that she receives the patent and begins the first day of the next part of her life.

Meanwhile, downstairs, her mother called the pawnshop asking about the price of the necklace. She was told that they were selling the necklace for $4000 and could not offer it for a lower price. Angela transferred $4000 from her savings account to her checking account, wrote a check for $4000 to the pawn shop, and went to the pawn shop the very next morning.

9
THE CAPGRAS DELUSION

In this chapter, we will review four cases of individuals whom we treated in our outpatient clinics over our careers and exhibited symptoms consistent with four of the most uncommon, and also most interesting, types of delusional beliefs: Capgras, Cotard, Folie à deux, and Fregoli.

"William" was a 65-year-old man with schizophrenia whom we had been treating in our clinic for several decades. He had developed schizophrenia in his early twenties while in the army and suffered primarily from relatively typical persecutory delusions and hallucinations. He was originally diagnosed with the paranoid type of schizophrenia given his substantial positive symptoms, mostly preserved affect, and limited negative symptoms and cognitive deficits. He never married. He was supported by disability and worked part-time in small restaurants as a chef. He was very happy with where he was in his life and considered himself to have dealt well with his diagnosis. He had been religiously taking 2mg of haloperidol every day for almost four decades. He had friends, was close with his family, and walked three miles every day. William was well known to our staff and was pleasant to everyone. He would often tell jokes during his session.

Over the previous several months, William had mentioned that he had noticed that his tongue would sometimes twitch and squirm and that his lips moved even when he did not mean for them to move. He indicated that he first noticed this while looking in the mirror and then paid more attention when his nephew asked him about the movements. William was able to suppress the movements on command, but they would generally begin again when he was not paying attention. They were neither painful nor bothersome, except when in public, although most people would have been unlikely to notice them.

During one of our routine sessions, William asked about these movements, which we had also noticed. It seemed clear that William was suffering from a mild form of tardive dyskinesia. Tardive dyskinesia is the most chronic or "tardive" occurring of the extrapyramidal side effects of antipsychotic medications, especially the so-called first-generation antipsychotic medications, such as haloperidol and fluphenazine. It tends to occur on a timescale of months to years. It is most associated with first-generation antipsychotic medications and especially those with the highest potency (i.e., those that require the lowest doses to be effective such as haloperidol and fluphenazine, whereas the risk is lower with medications such as chlorpromazine or thioridazine). It typically involves involuntary, irregular jerky movements of the face, tongue, or lips, and, in more severe forms, can include very high amplitude, incapacitating movements of the limbs and torso. Such severe forms of tardive dyskinesia, which could leave people bedbound due to inability to control their body, are rarely seen anymore since the advent of new, "second-generation" antipsychotic medications, which have less liability for extrapyramidal side effects and because psychiatrists are now aware that they do not have to use the very high doses of antipsychotic medications that people used to use. Tardive dyskinesia can become worse, remit, or remain stable. Sometimes increasing the dose of the current antipsychotic medication can result in temporary improvements. The best treatment and prevention are the use of the lowest possible doses of antipsychotic medications and to avoid high-potency first-generation agents.

We discussed all the options with William. He indicated that he definitely did not want to experience a return of his psychotic symptoms, but was also very distressed by his tardive dyskinesia. Therefore, William chose to switch medications to quetiapine, a second-generation antipsychotic medication with little to no liability for extrapyramidal side effects.

We cross-titrated William's medications over 16 weeks, given how long he had been taking haloperidol. He initially experienced no change in his symptoms or tardive dyskinesia. However, after titrating to 0.25mg haloperidol, he began to notice that his lip and tongue movements were decreasing in intensity. William was very pleased by this and, without consulting his psychiatrist, stopped taking haloperidol at all, several weeks before he and his psychiatrist had agreed upon.

William's next appointment was four weeks later. His tardive movements were nearly nonexistent, though William was not interested in talking about his movements. Rather, William described to his psychiatrist that one of the sous chefs at his place of employment was actually his commanding officer from the military. William reported feeling perplexed by how he did not realize it before, but was concerned that his commanding officer knew of his diagnosis of schizophrenia and was going to send a report to the army recommending that his honorable discharge be changed to a dishonorable discharge. After a long therapy session, it appeared that William had 100% conviction about this delusion, otherwise known as a Capgras delusion – namely, that someone close to a patient has been replaced by an impostor.

Fortunately, this delusion had not yet had too great of an effect on William and, despite having full conviction about the delusion, he was willing to wait to do anything until trying one or two other medications. Over the next six weeks we tried full doses of olanzapine and aripiprazole, with no change in his delusions. At this point, William and his psychiatrist made the decision to try haloperidol again, given that his delusion was refractory to other medications. He understood the risk of a return of his tardive dyskinesia and consented to the medication. We agreed to try a lower dose of haloperidol and titrated him to 0.5mg daily. Given anecdotal evidence that vitamin E can help with tardive dyskinesia, we also began prophylactic vitamin E supplementation. Within three days, William's Capgras delusion had all but remitted. Very low amplitude dyskinesias of his tongue and lips returned, but to a much lower degree than when he first experienced them. William continued 0.5mg haloperidol daily for several months with full resolution of his symptoms. His tardive dyskinesia remained minimal and stable, almost unrecognizable by the untrained observer. William was happy that he had recovered and was on a lower dose of haloperidol.

William's case of tardive dyskinesia is relatively typical. His decades of use of a high-potency first-generation antipsychotic medication likely contributed to his development of tardive dyskinesia. His ability to respond to a lower dose of haloperidol was probably related to the fact that, more than 40 years after his diagnosis, he had substantially lower body weight and had a less active condition (i.e., he was in the "residual" phase of the illness). Fortunately, with the advent of the newer antipsychotic medications and the understanding that most people with schizophrenia respond well to lower doses of antipsychotic medications (1), most trainees in mental health fields rarely come into contact with individuals with tardive dyskinesia.

"Judith" was a 29-year-old married, Asian-American female journalist who was recently discharged from a psychiatric hospital for a relapse of her schizophrenia. She had been diagnosed with schizophrenia when she was 20 years old during her index hospitalization. Her symptoms included delusions, hallucinations, negative symptoms, and, when at her worst, marked disorganization. Her course was typified by several years of stability followed by a relapse, during which she would invariably require hospitalization and a change in her medication regimen. Her medication adherence was very good. It was not completely understood why she would relapse while on full doses of her medications. She had previously responded to, and relapsed on, aripiprazole, risperidone, haloperidol, and olanzapine. She most recently relapsed while on full doses of lurasidone. During her most recent psychotic relapse, she experienced her typical symptoms – namely, disorganization, delusions, and hallucinations. Her disorganization was often manifest by derailing speech, during which she would speak with little focus, ending up on a topic unrelated to the topic on which she started. At her worst, her hygiene would suffer, so that she would stop showering or brushing her teeth or hair, and, at times, soil herself. Her delusions and hallucinations were bizarre in nature and often involved the belief that aliens were communicating with her. However, this time, she had developed a new theme to her delusions. In particular, she began to think that aliens from Mars were communicating with an agent from NASA who would serve as their liaison on Earth. She believed that they gave him the power to appear as different people, including people familiar to Judith, even though they were all really just the NASA agent. She described that the NASA agent was always inhabiting these other people and they all looked like their unique selves on the outside, but were actually just the NASA agent.

Judith was experiencing a Fregoli delusion. This is a rare and bizarre delusion in which a patient believes that a number of different people are actually just one person. It may occur along with a Capgras delusion, but may also occur on its own. It can be seen in individuals with schizophrenia, as well as in individuals with brain injury or other non-psychiatric conditions (e.g., medication-induced psychosis).

Judith's husband and parents were well aware of her symptoms, though were disturbed by how bizarre her newest delusion was. They quickly realized that she was experiencing a relapse. Upon recognizing these symptoms, they brought her to the emergency room, from where she was admitted to the inpatient psychiatric unit. On the inpatient psychiatric unit, Judith was placed on clozapine, given that she had become psychotic on full doses of five previous antipsychotic medications. She fully remitted within three weeks and was discharged home. She was sent to our outpatient clinic, rather than return to her previous clinic, because of our experience with clozapine.

Judith was a thin, well-dressed, young-appearing lady. She wore light-makeup and a recognizably expensive scent. She explained that she was very happy that clozapine had treated her symptoms. She was not bothered by the weekly blood draws, nor the risk of agranulocytosis, sialorrhea, or myocarditis. She understood how severe her condition was and that it was necessary to take medications. She reported that she was actually happy to be on clozapine as she was aware that it is the best antipsychotic medication for someone like her who could only maintain remission for several years at a time on other antipsychotic medications. She reported that each psychotic break was more and more intrusive to her life and she was hopeful that clozapine would allow her to maintain her remitted state.

What Judith was worried about, however, was the potential weight gain associated with clozapine. Judith was well aware of the risk of cardiometabolic side effects of antipsychotic medications and knew that clozapine has the greatest liability for these side effects (2). When people describe cardiometabolic side effects, they are primarily referring to weight gain, followed by dyslipidemia (primarily an increase in triglycerides), and then dysglycemia (increased insulin resistance, occasionally resulting in frank diabetes).

While second-generation antipsychotic medications tend to have less extra-pyramidal side effects than first-generation antipsychotic medications, they, as a group, have a greater liability for cardiometabolic side effects. First-generation antipsychotic medications also have a liability for cardiometabolic side effects, in particular the lower potency medications (i.e., those that require the highest doses to be effective such as chlorpromazine, whereas the risk is lower with medications such as haloperidol or fluphenazine), though overall this liability is less than with second-generation antipsychotic medications (2). In addition, among the second-generation antipsychotic medications, clozapine tends to have the highest liability, followed by olanzapine, quetiapine and risperidone, lurasidone and others.

Judith wanted to avoid weight gain at all costs. She explained that, as a journalist who spent substantial amounts of time on the air, it could be detrimental to her career to change in appearance in a significant way. She reported that she had gained five pounds on olanzapine and was aware that clozapine could cause more weight gain. She was willing to do whatever could be done to avoid weight gain, short of stop clozapine. She reported that she ate a very healthy, vegetarian diet, did not like sugary foods, and exercised six times a week. However, diabetes and weight gain were common in her family and she knew she was at high risk for both.

Judith was interested in potential medication approaches to minimizing weight gain associated with medications such as clozapine, such as topiramate and metformin (3). After discussing the advantages and disadvantages of each, including that the literature for metformin is strongest, she chose to add metformin 500mg twice daily to her clozapine. Judith experienced mild to moderate stomach upset upon starting metformin, but otherwise tolerated it very well. Five years after she began metformin and clozapine, she had still not gained any weight and remained fully remitted.

"Sid" was a 50-year-old married African American male with a history of schizophrenia. He had been diagnosed with schizophrenia 25 years prior and had been stably treated on one medication ever since. Sid was high functioning. He graduated college with a degree in Economics and graduate school with a Master's degree in accounting. He had been working as an accountant in private practice since he received his Master's degree. We had been seeing Sid in our clinic for ten years, approximately every three months. During the time that Sid was in our clinic, he had never experienced a relapse, was extremely medication adherent, and never missed an appointment.

One day in the early Spring, Sid came to our clinic for his appointment with his wife, "Charlene." This was notable because Sid usually came to his appointments alone. Sid and Charlene explained that things were going very well. Their daughter, "Gloria," had recently become engaged and their son, Isaiah, had graduated college and been admitted to medical school. They did, however, want to discuss that their pharmacist recently told them that the manufacturer of Sid's antipsychotic medication had recently decided to discontinue its production. They were worried what that meant for Sid's treatment, given that he had been so successfully and stably treated with this medication for so long. After confirming that the medication would no longer be available in any form, we discussed options, including trying a second-generation agent or other first-generation agents. Sid and Charlene explained that they were quite worried about a return of Sid's delusions and hallucinations and wanted to try whatever medication was most like his current medication. They understood that there were much newer and potentially safer medications available, but more than anything just wanted to maintain the status quo, given how severe positive symptoms can be. Therefore, they chose to try haloperidol, given how similar it is to his medication. They were aware of the potential side effects and consented to the medication.

Sid conducted his cross-titration from his medication to haloperidol over a two-month period, as he had two months of his medication left. He was able to tolerate a 5mg dose of haloperidol well. However, six weeks into his titration he began to report feelings of depression and that his internal gastrointestinal organs, including his intestines, liver, stomach, pancreas, and spleen, were rotting inside of him. He suggested that he would no longer exist within several weeks and was "essentially a corpse." Therefore, we increased his dose of haloperidol to 7.5mg and scheduled an appointment for one week later. At this point, he was noticeably anergic, apathetic, unemotional, and amotivated. He began missing work, sleeping all day, and disengaging from his life. He exhibited a paucity of thought and, when he would say something, perseverated on his death and non-existence. His wife reported that he was not showering, would eat only one meal a day, and moved at half of the pace at which he would usually move. She described that Sid was cooperative but would mostly just sleep all day or sit on the couch and do nothing except stare at walls. According to Charlene, Sid appeared "dead inside."

Sid had developed a Cotard delusion, which is the belief that one is dead or dying or that parts of one's body are decaying. Patients with this delusion may feel that they are dead, or feel immortal, albeit physically rotting and dead. Depressive symptoms are commonly a significant part of the clinical syndrome.

We decided to further increase Sid's haloperidol to 10mg daily and added an antidepressant, sertraline. We scheduled weekly appointments while Sid was in his current condition. At the next week's appointment, we noticed that Sid still endorsed his delusions of being dead and rotting inside, but with much less intensity than before. In addition, he had begun to speak, eat, and clean himself more. Sid continued to improve over the following three weeks, so that by four weeks from his last dose increase and the addition of sertraline, he was no longer endorsing delusions, was hygiening himself, and wanted to go back to work. Sid and Charlene were happy with Sid's improvement.

However, Sid still displayed much less affect than usual and moved more slowly than was typical for him. He had a festinating gate and would occasionally leave his mouth slightly open, allowing saliva to drip onto his shirt. He developed a moderately paced tremor in his right hand. He also fell down the stairs in their building. Sid and Charlene did not want to complain and were grateful that Sid's depression and delusions had resolved, but had questions about these persistent symptoms. Were these symptoms part of Sid's psychosis or part of his depression? Was it possible that Sid had developed negative symptoms this late into his condition?

The answer was neither of these three. Rather, Sid had developed parkinsonism, a sub-acute, extrapyramidal side effect of antipsychotic medications, especially the first-generation antipsychotic medications, such as haloperidol and fluphenazine. It tends to occur on a timescale of weeks to months. It is most associated with first-generation antipsychotic medications, and especially those with the highest potency (i.e., those that require the lowest doses to be effective such as haloperidol and fluphenazine, whereas the risk is lower with medications such as chlorpromazine or thioridazine). It typically involves symptoms that are seen in Parkinson's disease (hence the name), such as bradykinesia, postural instability, stiffness, and a pill-rolling tremor. These symptoms can often be mistaken for depression or negative symptoms and it can be hard to distinguish between them.

While parkinsonism is not always treatable, anticholinergic agents, such as benztropine and trihexyphenidyl, as well as dopaminergic agonists such as amantadine, have been known to help some patients with this side effect. The most effective intervention, however, is to decrease the dose of the offending medication, or switch to another agent with less liability for extrapyramidal side effects. We offered Sid and Charlene these options. They reported that their ideal situation would be to continue on haloperidol and take another medication, so they tried amantadine, which, fortunately had an almost immediate effect. By the next appointment, Sid's side effects had almost completely resolved. He and Charlene were happy with their new regimen and mentioned, as they left the office, that they hoped that the manufacturer of haloperidol would not stop producing it.

"Ms. Wagner" was a 49-year-old, widowed, Caucasian female who lived in a very small town in upstate New York. She lived with her 21-year-old daughter, "Harper," who was unmarried and worked as a waitress. Ms. Wagner had a 10th grade education. Her deceased husband, Mr. Wagner, was a truck driver and died after his truck was hit by a drunk driver, causing a severe and deadly collision. He died when Harper was only 2 years old. After his death, Ms. Wagner developed schizophrenia and required hospitalization. Her positive symptoms, primarily consisting of persecutory delusions about random people in the street wanting to kill her, waxed and waned since that time, mostly depending on whether or not she was taking her psychiatric medications. Ms. Wagner also had baseline negative symptoms that affected her energy level and motivation. She had been supported by social security since her diagnosis. In addition, since Harper turned 18 years old, she had been working and helping to support her mother. Ms. Wagner and Harper were very close. They had no other family in the area as Ms. Wagner was an only child and both her parents had died several years prior. Harper had several friends from her childhood, all of whom still lived in the area and were married with children. They had little time to spend with Harper. They would occasionally see each other in church or at the local grocery store, but otherwise had little interaction.

We met Ms. Wagner when her daughter brought her to our institution for an evaluation. Their neighborhood primary care physician had recently died and the new physician was not comfortable prescribing medications for schizophrenia. A recent graduate from one of our institution's medical training programs, he recommended that Ms. Wagner receive her care at our adult psychiatry resident clinic. She began treatment with a resident, under our supervision.

Approximately four months after she began her treatment in our resident's clinic, Ms. Wagner began to tell her resident that her neighbors were practicing witchcraft and sorcery and casting spells on her. The resident, who was understandably trying to impress us with descriptions of his thoroughness, explained to us that he was aware that certain religions, including the one to which Ms. Wagner belonged, believe in magic and witchcraft. We explained that, given how bizarre the delusion was, we did not think that Ms. Wagner's religion would have condoned such a belief, and since Ms. Wagner already had a diagnosis of schizophrenia, it was more likely that she had relapsed and was simply delusional. However, we encouraged the resident's careful approach and consideration of cultural differences and asked him to confirm for us the situation by obtaining collateral information from Ms. Wagner's daughter. Therefore, with Ms. Wagner's consent, the resident reached out to Harper for collateral information. Five minutes later, the resident, appearing very confident and happy, proclaimed that he was right. Harper had confirmed that what her mother was reporting was true and that she was also concerned about the neighbors. According to the resident, Harper explained that the neighbors were known to "dabble" in witchcraft, wizardry, enchantment, and clairvoyance and had decided to target Ms. Wagner and her mother because they were jealous that they still had a car, while the neighbors' car had been repossessed after they defaulted on their payments.

Finding it hard to believe that this story was not a delusion, we suggested that the resident make one last call to the new primary care physician in Ms. Wagner's town to obtain further collateral history as, 1) the physician lived in the town and would likely have known if something such as witchcraft were going on, and 2) the physician belonged to the same religion as did Ms. Wagner and her daughter and could therefore confirm whether or not these sorts of ideas were normal in their religion. Begrudgingly, the resident agreed to call the physician. He obtained consent from Ms. Wagner and spoke with the primary care physician. To the resident's great surprise, the primary care physician reported that he was unaware of anyone in the town engaging in, or having every engaged in, any sort of magic or witchcraft. The primary care physician also reported that witchcraft was not consistent in any way with their religious beliefs and that anyone in their community who believed in such a thing would likely be psychotic.

The resident reported this information to us and confessed that he did not understand what was happening. Together, we considered the possibility of folie à deux. Folie à deux is when a delusional belief held by one person is shared by another person. This can occur in individuals who are relatively isolated and close, such as in the case of Ms. Wagner and her daughter. The definitive test and treatment are separation for the person receiving the delusion and antipsychotic medications for the person originating the delusion.

We discussed our impression with Ms. Wagner and her daughter. Ms. Wagner agreed to admit herself into our inpatient psychiatric unit for further evaluation and treatment. Her dose of medication was doubled and within four days her delusion had resolved. Similarly, Harper, who came to pick Ms. Wagner up from the hospital seven days later, was no longer reporting any delusions.

Ms. Wagner continued to receive treatment in our clinic for many years thereafter. She remained stable and had no further relapses. Harper never demonstrated any other signs of psychosis, confirming our diagnosis of folie à deux. Harper eventually married a young man whom she met in the waiting area of our clinic while they were both accompanying their parents for visits with their psychiatrists. She quickly became pregnant and asked her mother to move in with her to help take care of her child. By all accounts, Ms. Wagner and Harper were living very fulfilling lives, free from witchcraft, sorcery, and magic, while full of reality and happiness.

References

1. McEvoy JP, Hogarty GE, Steingard S. Optimal dose of neuroleptic in acute schizophrenia. A controlled study of the neuroleptic threshold and higher haloperidol dose. *Arch Gen Psychiatry*. 1991;48(8):739–745.
2. Allison DB, Casey DE. Antipsychotic-induced weight gain: a review of the literature. *J Clin Psychiatry*. 2001;62 Suppl 7:22–31.
3. Mizuno Y, Suzuki T, Nakagawa A, Yoshida K, Mimura M, Fleischhacker WW, Uchida H. Pharmacological strategies to counteract antipsychotic-induced weight gain and metabolic adverse effects in schizophrenia: a systematic review and meta-analysis. *Schizophr Bull*. 2014;40(6):1385–1403.

10

VIOLENCE IN SCHIZOPHRENIA

The third year of medical school is when all medical students begin their clinical clerkships. That is, they spend about a month on a, usually, inpatient service for each of the major areas of medicine. It was on my Psychiatry rotation when two very important things happened. Both would affect my life for decades to come. The first was that it was during this rotation when my interest in Psychiatry was confirmed and I decided to pursue Psychiatry as a career. The second was that I came into contact with a patient named Jennifer.

"Jennifer" was a 27-year-old Caucasian female with schizophrenia. She came from a wealthy family of venture capitalists. Jennifer grew up in luxury, having numerous homes, vacation homes, luxury vehicles, and designer clothing. Her mother's jewelry collection alone was worth $10,000,000 and Jennifer's worth was already at least $5,000,000. Jennifer received the best and most expensive education at leading high schools in New York City and received an Ivy League college education. Upon graduation from college, she took a position in her father's firm. Approximately six months after she began working, she started to use marijuana, first on weekends, and then daily. Within four months, she had developed numerous delusions about being spied on by other venture capital firms and the Securities and Exchange Commission (SEC). She was also experiencing frank auditory hallucinations of the same nature – namely, voices that she thought were from people in the SEC and other venture capital firms suggesting that Jennifer's firm was engaged in illegal activities (which they were not). Jennifer's delusions and auditory hallucinations became very intense, worsened by her continued use of marijuana and lack of treatment. She was first hospitalized after she attacked an employee whom she thought was secretly working with the SEC with a knife. Jennifer was hospitalized for only five days as her condition quickly remitted with medications and abstinence from marijuana. She was discharged and resumed her life. While she was mostly able to remain abstinent from marijuana, Jennifer, due to a lack of insight, quickly stopped her medications and, after three months, was hospitalized again after being found screaming at someone on the street. Jennifer was again accusing this person of being secretly involved with the SEC.

This pattern continued for several years. Jennifer would quickly remit with medications, return home and to work, and then stop her medications, begin to experience delusions and hallucinations, become overtly hostile or violent, and require rehospitalization. I first came into contact with her five years into her illness, during one of her hospitalizations. She had been brought to the emergency room by the police after she grabbed the cellular phone of a bystander, whom she thought was surveilling her, and threw it into traffic.

At first, Jennifer developed a positive therapeutic alliance with me. As with her previous hospitalizations, she recovered very quickly on small doses of olanzapine. By her third day in the hospital, her psychotic symptoms had almost completely remitted. However, I found that there was more to Jennifer than her psychosis. I was struck by how poorly she would treat other staff members and patients, especially minorities. Most patients would politely ask the hospital staff for help, or medications, as they needed them. Jennifer, on the other hand, demanded things, and when she did not get her way, would begin to refer to someone in an obscene way, usually referring to the size of their genitalia if male, or, if a minority, to their race or ethnicity in some derogatory manner.

One day during our daily session, the psychology extern and I were discussing with Jennifer her recent behavior and how the attending physician had restricted her privileges due to her behavior. She was describing how she saw no reason for this and that the young lady with anorexia, whom she most recently made cry after calling her "fat and ugly" and telling her that "it's no wonder that your fiancé left you," was just "emotionally weak and dumb" and that I was "the only one smart enough to understand someone of her caliber." The psychology extern then suggested to Jennifer that maybe the attending physician restricted her privileges for a reason, perhaps to allow her time to reflect on more adaptive ways to interact with people. Jennifer became quiet and thoughtful. The psychology extern noticed that his observation had elicited the intended response. Therefore, perhaps prematurely, he continued with an interpretation. He said, "Is it possible that you call people names and treat them like they are less valuable than you are, not because of what you really think about them, but because you actually feel that YOU do not have much value. This feeling is too difficult for you to deal with, so you project it onto other people rather than deal with your feelings of inadequacy about yourself."

In all my decades of work with psychiatric patients I have never seen a therapeutic intervention so poorly timed and, as a consequence, receive so absolute and definitive a response. Jennifer went from being thoughtful to cunningly smiling, and then began a five minute, expletive-laden roast of the psychology extern, attacking everything about him, including, but not limited to, his height (he was about five feet, seven inches tall), his need for glasses, his very slight Midwestern accent, his olive-colored skin, his seven syllable name, the fact that he was a psychologist in training, his "ugly" wife (Jennifer actually had no idea what his wife looked like, but assumed based on the appearance of the psychology extern, according to her), the mole on his right cheek, his voice which would occasionally crack, that he was receiving his education at a public university, his attire, and many more characteristics, real or fake, that are too numerous to mention or remember. After five minutes of this, it became clear that Jennifer was getting under the extern's skin. He was too hurt to say anything. I interrupted the session and walked the psychology extern back to the nurse's station. Jennifer was discharged later that day to the delight of both the patients and staff on the unit and especially to the delight of the psychology extern, from whom I never heard again.

I did, however, hear from Jennifer again, not long after I finished my rotation on the inpatient unit. It started with angry phone calls, about 15 voicemail messages over the next year, primarily derogatory in nature, similar to the language that she used to denigrate people on the unit, making fun of my appearance, name, education, etc. Though bothersome, I was informed that no real crime was being committed, besides harassment, which was, in the opinion of those from whom I was obtaining guidance, not worth the effort to pursue. I was told that I should just try to "ignore" the calls.

Unfortunately, the nature of the calls became more serious and more psychotic. It appeared that, as per her pattern, Jennifer had stopped her medications and incorporated me into her delusional system. On my voicemail, I began to receive messages from Jennifer saying that she had caught on to what my colleagues and I were really trying to do, which was to lock her up in prison for insider trading, avoiding federal income and corporate taxes, and killing her optometrist. I shared all this information with law enforcement and appropriate administrative personnel who examined the claims and found that none of them were true. In fact, Jennifer, because of her now persistent psychosis (due to not taking medications), was no longer working and no longer living with her parents. Law enforcement did report that her optometrist had recently died, though there were no reports of, or evidence suggesting, foul play or intentional death.

The calls continued, with similar content to the messages she had previously left. Then, one day, she showed up at my gym. Over the next several weeks she showed up several more times. She initially did not acknowledge me or try to come near me. The fourth time she appeared at my gym, however, was different. She was belligerent and hostile. She approached me while I was lifting weights and began yelling at me, blaming me for her diagnosis of schizophrenia, saying that I was a bad psychiatrist and telling me to stop monitoring her. Fortunately, the gym owner explained to Jennifer that she would have to leave the gym if she could not settle down. When she began to yell at him, he informed Jennifer that if she did not leave the gym he would call the police. She left shortly thereafter and did not return to the gym.

The voicemail messages continued for several more years, although, fortunately, there were no more sightings of Jennifer. The messages tended to worsen every time a noteworthy or prominent businessman was indicted for fraud or insider trading. The calls peaked after one very prominent example, after which Jennifer left a message indicating that she was going to kill me.

We immediately called law enforcement. Initially attentive, they suggested that this was very serious. However, once we gave information about ourselves and Jennifer, namely that we were psychiatrists and that Jennifer was a patient with schizophrenia, they paused, chuckled, and said that they were very busy and did not have the time to look into every "silly thing that crazy people say to their psychiatrists."

Dangerousness in psychotic individuals is a very serious and important topic. While the vast majority of psychotic people are not dangerous, and most violence is committed by non-psychotic people (1), there are data that suggest a link between psychosis and violence. Overall, almost 10%–30% of individuals with psychosis are violent over a six-month period (2–6), though the vast majority of this risk is related to substance use (7). This work and others has led some to suggest a link between violence and psychosis (8).

Further, aggression is associated with worse outcome in schizophrenia (9) and the link between violence and mental illness contributes to stigma (10). Finally, the consequences of violence, such as incarceration, hospitalization, and victimization further add to the stigma experienced by individuals with psychosis (11). Therefore, decreasing violence risk in psychosis is clinically relevant and has important public health implications.

Therefore, substantial effort has been directed toward understanding the risk factors for violence among psychotic individuals. These include a history of violence, positive symptoms (12–22), especially command hallucinations and persecutory delusions, non-adherence with medications (23, 24), poor insight (25), alcohol and substance use (26–30), antisocial conduct (31), stressful life circumstances and environment (32), traumatic brain injury (33), impulsivity (34, 35), and cognitive deficits (36, 37). Negative symptoms tend to be protective (5).

Some individuals consider violence in psychosis to have three main mechanisms through which all other mediating and moderating factors work: impulsivity, psychopathy, and positive symptoms (38, 39). So, for example, drug use would increase risk for violence via effects on impulsivity and positive symptoms, traumatic brain injury via effects on impulsivity, etc.

While understanding risk factors and mechanisms for violence in psychosis are helpful, it has not allowed the field to progress to the point where we can reliably or accurately predict violence or prevent violence. Antipsychotic medications, and particularly clozapine, are thought to decrease risk for violence (6, 23, 24, 40–44), although the mechanisms by which they work remain elusive.

Work by our group is shedding new light on our understanding of violence in psychosis, with a novel focus on violent ideation. In a recent longitudinal study, we measured violent ideation and violent behavior in 200 individuals at clinical high-risk for psychosis (45). Patients were then followed for two years and were assessed for outcome violent behavior, as well as conversion to psychosis. We found that baseline violent ideation and violent behavior predicted both outcome violent behavior as well as conversion to psychosis, independent of all clinical and demographic variables. In addition, the time between the outcome violent behavior and the conversion to psychosis over the whole two-year period was, amazingly, on average only seven days. We further examined what questions elicited violent ideation at baseline and found that questions that directly ask about violent thoughts, such as "Have you had thoughts of harming anyone else?" elicited no violent ideation, while other questions, such as questions about intrusive, ego-dystonic thoughts, did. Finally, we found that none of the targets of the outcome violent behavior were the same as the targets that were initially identified at baseline, indicating that the targets changed over time.

Further, in an effort to better understand the neurobiology of violent ideation in individuals at clinical high-risk for psychosis, we examined the amygdala of 70 individuals, 21 with violent ideation and 49 without violent ideation (46). We found that those with violent ideation had abnormal and asymmetric amygdalar volumes. These findings suggest similarities in the pathogenesis of violence in psychiatric patients, as well as that there may be both phenomenological and neurobiological links between psychosis and violence.

Our findings, considered with other work on violence in psychosis, allowed us to propose a model for psychosis in violence (47). This model suggests that violent thoughts are common, intrusive, and ego-dystonic in the prodromal or clinical high-risk period when the risk for violence is low. However, with the first-episode of psychosis comes a breakdown in inhibitions, organization, and executive control that leads to a period of peak risk for violence. With treatment, hospitalization, and resolution of the first-episode, the risk of violence decreases substantially to near background levels. Risk for violence rises during periods of non-adherence with medications, substance use, and inpatient hospitalization.

While these findings, and our model, are helpful, we remain very far from understanding violence in psychosis well enough to claim an ability to accurately predict it, which is the ultimate goal. The next step would be the development of an instrument capable of identifying individuals at high-risk for violence without over identifying people not at risk (false positives) or under identifying people at risk (false negatives). For this, we believe that focusing on violent ideation, in addition to risk factors, will provide the extra accuracy we need to achieve our goals.

However, studies of violence in psychosis are very hard to implement for a number of reasons, including the very low prevalence of violence in psychotic individuals. However, we have found that perhaps the greatest impediments to this work on violence in psychosis are stigma and overprotectiveness. Many very well-meaning psychiatrists, psychologists, and mental health advocates resist any attempt to suggest a link, however small, between psychosis and violence.

Yet, we, as a society, are bombarded by the reality that psychotic individuals are overrepresented among perpetrators of mass violence, and by the scientific evidence, as summarized above, linking violence to psychosis.

Therefore, studying, speaking about, and writing about violence in psychosis are challenging. However, we are up to this challenge, and feel that, rather than stigmatize individuals with psychosis, studying violent ideas and behaviors in psychosis reduces stigma. One way to think about this is to consider suicide in depression. Until *recently* (we place asterisks here to include the caveat that suicidality remains a very stigmatized subject, though society is in a better place now than where we were a few decades ago) suicidality was very stigmatizing, so much so that providers and patients alike would not talk about it, due to patients' concerns of being "crazy," or clinicians' concerns about extra effort/litigation etc. However, suicidal ideation is common and an inherent, though not pervasive, part of depression. Suicidal ideation can be passive (ego dystonic) or active (ego syntonic). More severe suicidality implies worse illness. Asking about suicide does not cause suicide.

When we talk or write about violence in psychosis, after clarifying that most psychotic people are not violent and that most violence is not perpetrated by psychotic people, we recommend that people exchange "violence" for "suicide" and "psychosis" for "depression." That would result in the following statements: Violence is very stigmatizing, so much so that providers and patients alike do not talk about it, due to patients' concerns of being "crazy," or clinicians' concerns about extra effort/litigation etc. However, violent ideation is common and an inherent, though not pervasive, part of psychosis. Violent ideation can be passive (ego dystonic) or active (ego syntonic). More severe violence implies worse illness. Asking about violence does not cause violence.

Our ultimate goals are to: 1) decrease the stigma that patients now feel about discussing violent thoughts, which are common in psychotic people, with providers; 2) develop accurate and practical violence risk assessment instruments; and 3) understand the mechanisms by which medications such as clozapine and other antipsychotic medications decrease risk for violence. Realizing these goals would have great and positive implications for society as a whole, for the field of psychiatry, and for people such as Jennifer.

References

1. Taylor PJ. Psychosis and violence: stories, fears, and reality. *Can J Psychiatry*. 2008;53(10):647–659.
2. Joyal CC, Gendron C, Cote G. Nature and frequency of aggressive behaviours among long-term inpatients with schizophrenia: a 6-month report using the modified overt aggression scale. *Can J Psychiatry*. 2008;53(7):478–481.
3. Large MM, Nielssen O. Violence in first-episode psychosis: a systematic review and meta-analysis. *Schizophr Res*. 2011;125(2–3):209–220.

4. Steadman HJ, Mulvey EP, Monahan J, Robbins PC, Appelbaum PS, Grisso T, Roth LH, Silver E. Violence by people discharged from acute psychiatric inpatient facilities and by others in the same neighborhoods. *Arch Gen Psychiatry*. 1998;55(5):393–401.

5. Swanson JW, Swartz MS, Van Dorn RA, Elbogen EB, Wagner HR, Rosenheck RA, Stroup TS, McEvoy JP, Lieberman JA. A national study of violent behavior in persons with schizophrenia. *Arch Gen Psychiatry*. 2006;63(5):490–499.

6. Swanson JW, Swartz MS, Van Dorn RA, Volavka J, Monahan J, Stroup TS, McEvoy JP, Wagner HR, Elbogen EB, Lieberman JA. Comparison of antipsychotic medication effects on reducing violence in people with schizophrenia. *Br J Psychiatry*. 2008;193(1):37–43.

7. Fazel S, Gulati G, Linsell L, Geddes JR, Grann M. Schizophrenia and violence: systematic review and meta-analysis. *PLoS Med*. 2009;6(8):e1000120.

8. Walsh E, Buchanan A, Fahy T. Violence and schizophrenia: examining the evidence. *Br J Psychiatry*. 2002;180:490–495.

9. Shrivastava A, Shah N, Johnston M, Stitt L, Thakar M. Predictors of long-term outcome of first-episode schizophrenia: a ten-year follow-up study. *Indian J Psychiatry*. 2010;52(4):320–326.

10. Phelan JC, Link BG. The growing belief that people with mental illnesses are violent: the role of the dangerousness criterion for civil commitment. *Soc Psychiatry Psychiatr Epidemiol*. 1998;33 Suppl 1:S7–S12.

11. Hodgins S. Violent behaviour among people with schizophrenia: a framework for investigations of causes, and effective treatment, and prevention. *Philos Trans R Soc Lond B, Biol Sci*. 2008;363(1503):2505–2518.

12. Lindqvist P, Allebeck P. Schizophrenia and crime. A longitudinal follow-up of 644 schizophrenics in Stockholm. *Br J Psychiatry*. 1990;157:345–350.

13. Hodgins S, Mednick SA, Brennan PA, Schulsinger F, Engberg M. Mental disorder and crime. Evidence from a Danish birth cohort. *Arch Gen Psychiatry*. 1996;53(6):489–496.

14. Swanson JW, Swartz MS, Essock SM, Osher FC, Wagner HR, Goodman LA, Rosenberg SD, Meador KG. The social-environmental context of violent behavior in persons treated for severe mental illness. *Am J Public Health*. 2002;92(9):1523–1531.

15. Taylor PJ, Bragado-Jimenez MD. Women, psychosis and violence. *Int J Law Psychiatry*. 2009;32(1):56–64.

16. Douglas KS, Guy LS, Hart SD. Psychosis as a risk factor for violence to others: a meta-analysis. *Psychol Bull*. 2009;135(5):679–706.

17. Bartels SJ, Drake RE, Wallach MA, Freeman DH. Characteristic hostility in schizophrenic outpatients. *Schizophr Bull*. 1991;17(1):163–171.

18. Taylor PJ, Leese M, Williams D, Butwell M, Daly R, Larkin E. Mental disorder and violence: a special (high security) hospital study. *Br J Psychiatry*. 1998;172:218–226.

19. McNiel DE, Eisner JP, Binder RL. The relationship between command hallucinations and violence. *Psychiatr Serv*. 2000;51(10):1288–1292.

20. Coid JW, Ullrich S, Kallis C, Keers R, Barker D, Cowden F, Stamps R. The relationship between delusions and violence: findings from the East London first episode psychosis study. *JAMA Psychiatry*. 2013;70(5):465–471.

21. Keers R, Ullrich S, Destavola BL, Coid JW. Association of violence with emergence of persecutory delusions in untreated schizophrenia. *Am J Psychiatry*. 2014;171(3):332–339.

22. Ullrich S, Keers R, Coid JW. Delusions, anger, and serious violence: new findings from the MacArthur Violence Risk Assessment Study. *Schizophr Bull*. 2014;40(5):1174–1181.

23. Yesavage JA. Inpatient violence and the schizophrenic patient: an inverse correlation between danger-related events and neuroleptic levels. *Biol Psychiatry*. 1982; 17(11):1331–1337.

24. Elbogen EB, Van Dorn RA, Swanson JW, Swartz MS, Monahan J. Treatment engagement and violence risk in mental disorders. *Br J Psychiatry*. 2006;189:354–360.

25. Buckley PF, Hrouda DR, Friedman L, Noffsinger SG, Resnick PJ, Camlin-Shingler K. Insight and its relationship to violent behavior in patients with schizophrenia. *Am J Psychiatry*. 2004;161(9):1712–1714.

26. Eronen M, Tiihonen J, Hakola P. Schizophrenia and homicidal behavior. *Schizophr Bull*. 1996;22(1):83–89.

27. Rasanen P, Tiihonen J, Isohanni M, Rantakallio P, Lehtonen J, Moring J. Schizophrenia, alcohol abuse, and violent behavior: a 26-year followup study of an unselected birth cohort. *Schizophr Bull*. 1998;24(3):437–441.

28. Swartz MS, Swanson JW, Hiday VA, Borum R, Wagner HR, Burns BJ. Violence and severe mental illness: the effects of substance abuse and nonadherence to medication. *Am J Psychiatry*. 1998;155(2):226–231.

29. Arseneault L, Moffitt TE, Caspi A, Taylor PJ, Silva PA. Mental disorders and violence in a total birth cohort: results from the Dunedin Study. *Arch Gen Psychiatry*. 2000;57(10):979–986.

30. Elbogen EB, Johnson SC. The intricate link between violence and mental disorder: results from the National Epidemiologic Survey on Alcohol and Related Conditions. *Arch Gen Psychiatry*. 2009;66(2):152–161.

31. Swanson JW, Van Dorn RA, Swartz MS, Smith A, Elbogen EB, Monahan J. Alternative pathways to violence in persons with schizophrenia: the role of childhood antisocial behavior problems. *Law Hum Behav*. 2008;32(3):228–240.

32. Volavka J, Citrome L. Pathways to aggression in schizophrenia affect results of treatment. *Schizophr Bull*. 2011;37(5):921–929.

33. Sariaslan A, Lichtenstein P, Larsson H, Fazel S. Triggers for violent criminality in patients with psychotic disorders. *JAMA Psychiatry*. 2016;73(8):796–803.

34. Krakowski MI, De Sanctis P, Foxe JJ, Hoptman MJ, Nolan K, Kamiel S, Czobor P. Disturbances in response inhibition and emotional processing as potential pathways to violence in schizophrenia: a high-density event-related potential study. *Schizophr Bull*. 2016;42(4):963–974.

35. Nolan KA, D'Angelo D, Hoptman MJ. Self-report and laboratory measures of impulsivity in patients with schizophrenia or schizoaffective disorder and healthy controls. *Psychiatry Res*. 2011;187(1–2):301–303.

36. Reinharth J, Reynolds G, Dill C, Serper M. Cognitive predictors of violence in schizophrenia: a meta-analytic review. *Schizophrenia Research: Cognition*. 2014;1:101–111.

37. Ahmed AO, Richardson J, Buckner A, Romanoff S, Feder M, Oragunye N, Ilnicki A, Bhat I, Hoptman MJ, Lindenmayer JP. Do cognitive deficits predict negative emotionality and aggression in schizophrenia? *Psychiatry Res*. 2018;259:350–357.

38. Stahl SM. Deconstructing violence as a medical syndrome: mapping psychotic, impulsive, and predatory subtypes to malfunctioning brain circuits. *CNS Spectr*. 2014;19(5):357–365.

39. Hoptman MJ. Impulsivity and aggression in schizophrenia: a neural circuitry perspective with implications for treatment. *CNS Spectr*. 2015;20(3):280–286.

40. Citrome L, Volavka J, Czobor P, Sheitman B, Lindenmayer JP, McEvoy J, Cooper TB, Chakos M, Lieberman JA. Effects of clozapine, olanzapine, risperidone, and haloperidol on hostility among patients with schizophrenia. *Psychiatr Serv*. 2001;52(11):1510–1514.

41. Volavka J, Czobor P, Nolan K, Sheitman B, Lindenmayer JP, Citrome L, McEvoy JP, Cooper TB, Lieberman JA. Overt aggression and psychotic symptoms in patients with schizophrenia treated with clozapine, olanzapine, risperidone, or haloperidol. *J Clin Psychopharmacol*. 2004;24(2):225–228.

42. Krakowski MI, Czobor P, Citrome L, Bark N, Cooper TB. Atypical antipsychotic agents in the treatment of violent patients with schizophrenia and schizoaffective disorder. *Arch Gen Psychiatry*. 2006;63(6):622–629.

43. Swanson JW, Swartz MS, Elbogen EB. Effectiveness of atypical antipsychotic medications in reducing violent behavior among persons with schizophrenia in community-based treatment. *Schizophr Bull*. 2004;30(1):3–20.

44. Buckley PF. The role of typical and atypical antipsychotic medications in the management of agitation and aggression. *J Clin Psychiatry*. 1999;60 (Suppl 10):52–60.

45. Brucato G, Appelbaum PS, Lieberman JA, Wall MM, Feng T, Masucci MD, Altschuler R, Girgis RR. A longitudinal study of violent behavior in a psychosis-risk cohort. *Neuropsychopharmacology*. 2018;43(2):264–271.

46. Feng X, Provenzano F, Appelbaum PS, Masucci MD, Brucato G, Lieberman JA, Girgis RR. Amygdalar volume and violent ideation in a sample at clinical high-risk for psychosis. *Psychiatry Res Neuroimaging*. 2019;287:60–62.

47. Brucato G, Appelbaum PS, Masucci MD , Rolin S, Wall MM, Levin M, Altschuler R, First MB, Lieberman JA, Girgis RR. Prevalence and phenomenology of violent ideation and behavior among 200 young people at clinical high-risk for psychosis: an emerging model of violence and psychotic illness. *Neuropsychopharmacology*. 2019;44(5):907–914.

11

AUDITORY HALLUCINATIONS AND RELIGIOUS DELUSIONS

"Remy" was a 50-year-old Spanish female, born in the 1960s and raised in the Valencia region of Spain. Her family, who were citrus farmers in a rural community, were devout Roman Catholics. Like most people in their region, they attended mass several times weekly. She, her parents, and a younger sister would recite the rosary upon awakening each morning, say grace before meals, and pray before retiring at night. In their living room they constructed a small shrine for a statue of the Blessed Virgin Mary, shown crushing the devil with her foot, and festooned with holy pictures and flowers. Most of the people with whom they would regularly interact were members of their church community and virtually everything that happened in their home and town was understood or explained in spiritual terms. For example, a good harvest was interpreted as a sign of approval from God, while a poor bounty suggested they had displeased Heaven in some way. The latter would prompt increased prayer and church attendance, personal penances, and supplications for forgiveness and mercy.

Remy was raised during the period of rapid economic and industrial growth in Spain from 1959 through 1974 known as the "Spanish Miracle." Unable to keep up with the technological advancements of government-aided farmers, Remy's family, like many traditional citrus farmers, were run out of business and left Spain for other countries. She and her family uprooted themselves and began life afresh in the United States – in a bustling, multicultural neighborhood in Queens, New York City.

Remy, who was 11 when she arrived in America, struggled to learn English and acclimatize to her new environment. She had always been somewhat shy and now felt especially uncomfortable making connections with new people. She passed most of her free time alone, reading books about history and religion. Her difficulties adapting to her new community were compounded by the fact that her family's culture was markedly different than that of her peers and their neighbors. For instance, she and her family wore the traditional garb of their area of Spain. For the first time, Remy was exposed to not only other sects of Christianity, but also entirely different faiths. Her classmates would ridicule her accent and clothes. Thus, Remy had a particularly lonely childhood.

Remy eventually became fluent in English. She began to do well in school and better understand the trends and fashions of her new community. In addition, Remy's family became friendly with a small group of other Catholic farmers from Valencia who had also immigrated to Queens. Remy and the other children from these families grew close and spent time together. They would also go to church together and participate in Bible study at each other's homes. Most of Remy's friends also attended high school together. Therefore, in high school, Remy felt less like an outsider. She earned good grades and, while still quiet and soft-spoken, she was much happier and more socially active than she had been since leaving Spain.

Remy went to college near her parents' home and lived at home throughout. It was expected in Remy's home that, as a woman, she would reside with her parents until she married. At no point did Remy consider doing otherwise as she enjoyed warm, supportive relationships with her parents. Remy graduated with a bachelor's degree in English as a second language and went on to work as an ESL teacher at a school in Manhattan. Around this time, many of her friends married and began having children. This led to Remy becoming isolated once again, but she relished this time alone. Besides going to work, she spent much time in church and attending Bible classes. The rest of her time was spent talking with her parents, praying, or reading spiritual books.

By the time Remy reached her late 20s her parents began to worry that she was still unmarried and showing no interest in finding a husband. She was speaking about becoming a nun. While an honorable life path, joining a convent did not seem, to her parents, to be Remy's true vocation. They encouraged Remy to hold out on her thoughts of entering a convent and to allow God to send her a good, Catholic man.

It seemed that the time had come two years later. Remy's priest approached her parents about a young man named Juan who had recently arrived from Valencia and had asked the priest if there were any unwed women from traditional families in the area. Juan was 30 years old, approximately one year older than Remy. He came from a similarly religious background and had relocated from Spain five years earlier. As he was one year away from completing his doctoral degree in physics, he felt it would be a good time to get married and start a family.

Remy's parents consented to Remy and Juan courting, and, within three months, they were married. The first nine years of their marriage were happy and uneventful. They had three children, all of whom were healthy, energetic, and well-behaved. They brought up their children in a robustly Catholic household and were highly involved with their church. Juan gradually worked his way up in the physics field and became quite successful, transitioning from academia to industry. Remy was a devoted homemaker. She was pleased that she had listened to her parents and waited for Juan to come into her life.

When Remy was 39, her beloved father suddenly succumbed to a heart attack. Remy was devastated. It was at this juncture that things began to change for Remy. She grew increasingly religious, spending three to four hours a day praying in her bedroom. She began making references to her mother and husband about a demonic entity being out to get her and her children. She hung crucifixes in every room of the house and on the front door. She felt that she was only safe from the demon in her home or at church so that, whenever she was elsewhere, she would repeatedly make the Sign of the Cross, irrespective of the setting. Although she never admitted to auditory hallucinations, she began to hear a low, sinister-sounding voice mocking her and condemning her and her family. She would randomly say "No!" in an effort to block these assertions. On one occasion, Remy's middle child found her in the garage, shouting and wildly gesturing in an effort to keep the entity from possessing her. When Remy saw her son, her manner abruptly changed and she calmly attended to him.

Remy also began to feel she could communicate directly with God. Beyond her usual prayer, Remy began to see communications from God in nearly everything around her, such as birdsong, weather patterns, and her children's grades at school. For instance, when her son brought home a report card with a grade of "B," she thought this was God's way of telling her he had been "bad" and had him pray for forgiveness. Beyond thinking, as was typical for her culture, that various events might reflect God's will, Remy began to talk about how God would communicate with her about future events, such as Juan having problems at work or her daughter being accepted into a prestigious club.

These signs persisted for several years. Although experiencing psychotic illness, Remy was, for the most part, able to function. She took care of her family and their finances and was typically able to conceal overtly bizarre behavior in church or when around other people, such as at the grocery store or bank. Although her family recognized that something was wrong, they had virtually no understanding of psychiatric illness, nor what to do to help.

On one occasion when Remy was 45 years old, she and her family went shopping at a mall. At the onset, the day was fairly unremarkable. Remy was generally paranoid and overly religious, making the Sign of the Cross countless times after they pulled their car out of the driveway. The family had learned to live with and accept this "habit." Today, however, would prove unique. After shopping for two hours, they were waiting in line at a cash register. Remy became acutely agitated and abruptly used her hand to strike the person behind her, accusing the stranger of being a demonic agent. Remy did not seriously injure the person, who was generally understanding when Juan explained that his wife was "not herself" and "going through something." Not knowing what else to do, Juan dropped the children off at home and took Remy to a local emergency room. At this point,

Remy was screaming and yelling about the demon she believed was seeking to destroy her and her family and that everyone outside of the church was part of this plan. She was overtly hallucinating and frequently responding to voices by shouting out, "No!"

In the emergency room, Remy's behavior rapidly deescalated with 5mg of olanzapine, commonly prescribed to acutely agitated and/or psychotic individuals in such settings. She underwent a basic medical work-up, as well as a magnetic resonance imaging (MRI) scan, to rule out any obvious brain abnormalities, of which there were none. Remy was diagnosed with schizophrenia, based on her behavior, years of experiencing the two positive symptoms of a religious delusion and auditory hallucinations, and lack of other potential causes, such as substance or alcohol use, or a medical condition. After several hours in the ER, Remy was now calm. She continued to endorse delusions as well was mild auditory hallucinations, but was in greater control of herself. She was discharged with a follow-up appointment to see a psychiatrist at a nearby outpatient clinic.

Over the next five years Remy saw several different providers. She continued to take olanzapine each night, although with varying degrees of adherence. At times, when she would take the medication less often, she would become noticeably more irritable and spend more time in prayer. Occasionally, she would be found in heated arguments with the demon she believed was in the room. These behaviors were generally very obvious to her husband and sometimes her children, who would then make sure that Remy was taking her medications as prescribed. Although Remy's insight into her condition was poor, she would usually comply with her family's wishes, thereby avoiding trips to the emergency room or psychiatric inpatient hospitalizations.

Remy's condition eventually became more stable, as is typical for individuals in the chronic phase of schizophrenia. Her delusions and hallucinations, while still present at baseline, became less severe and frequent, even when she had not taken her medication for several days. In addition, she began to develop mild negative symptoms and cognitive deficits. Remy's energy level began to decline, so that she would need to sleep nine or ten hours a day. With her children all in college, Remy would often spend hours on end sitting in a chair at home, staring at a wall. She remained appropriate and pleasant when outside or at church, but otherwise engaged in no social interactions. Her affect become more constricted, with less laughing and smiling. Overall, Remy's day consisted of waking up, drinking coffee, praying for several hours, reading a few pages of a spiritual book, running errands, preparing and eating dinner, cleaning up, and going to bed. On Sundays, she attended mass.

One day, Remy's older daughter noticed that her mother seemed less attentive than usual. She would occasionally ask her daughter to speak more slowly or to repeat herself. Frequently, her daughter would call for her mother who was just a few feet away and Remy did not respond. By this time, computers, the internet and smartphones were ubiquitous. Remy, however, was unable – or unwilling – to learn to use any of these technologies, despite her family's constant encouragement.

Remy's course of schizophrenia was typical in some ways and atypical in others. While the condition tends to affect females at a slightly later age than males, it is uncommon, although not rare, for it to begin in a woman's late 30s or early 40s. This is slightly more common, however, for people with the paranoid subtype of schizophrenia, as did Remy. Although the classification of schizophrenia into subtypes was discontinued with the transition to the fifth edition of the *Diagnostic and Statistical Manual of Mental Disorders* (DSM-5), published in 2013 (1), the prior edition delineated five subcategories (2). In the paranoid subtype, delusions and hallucinations are the predominant symptoms. Disorganization, negative symptoms and cognitive deficits may be present, but are usually not severe and may only mildly affect a person's functioning and capacity to live a reasonably normal life. Paranoid schizophrenia has the best long-term outcome among the different subtypes of schizophrenia and tends to have a later onset than other subtypes.

Disorganized schizophrenia, on the other hand, is characterized by marked disorganization of speech, behavior, and affect that leads to significant disability. This tends to occur earlier than other subtypes and carries a poor prognosis. People with disorganized schizophrenia are frequently hospitalized and make up a large proportion of chronically institutionalized persons. Individuals with disorganized schizophrenia may have delusions and hallucinations and will definitely demonstrate negative symptoms and cognitive deficits, although disorganization is the most prominent group of symptoms they will show. These individuals are often the ones that become disheveled, homeless, and transient. They may develop a very strong odor from not cleaning themselves and can be extremely hard to understand because of their disorganized speech. Types of disorganized speech include tangentiality, where there is poor focus to one's speech so that they never get back to the initial topic when speaking. In circumstantiality, one starts talking about something and eventually ends up back on that topic, but only after substantially unfocused speech. One may exhibit loosening of associations, in which one observes a sequence of disconnected or only remotely related ideas. Thought blocking occurs when someone is so disorganized that he or she cannot finish a thought and may stop speaking mid-sentence, or just not initiate a sentence at all. Sometimes, one's speech can become so unfocused and jumbled that it can be described as "word salad," such that there are no discernable links between the different words that someone is using, as if one is randomly reciting words out of a dictionary.

Catatonic schizophrenia is also quite severe. This subtype was far more common during the era before antipsychotic medications were in wide use. People whose symptoms meet criteria for this subtype demonstrate severe catatonia, which implies the maintenance of bizarre, peculiar postures for minutes, hours or even days at a time. Mutism is commonly observed in catatonic schizophrenia.

Alternatively, such persons may show excessive, disinhibited, and purposeless motor activity, such as constantly walking or jumping around, or moving different parts of the body without clear direction. Catatonic schizophrenia may be especially responsive to intravenous benzodiazepines, such as lorazepam, or to electroconvulsive therapy (ECT).

Undifferentiated schizophrenia is essentially an umbrella term for all other types of schizophrenia. This diagnosis is given when catatonia, disorganization, and paranoia are not the most prominent features of one's schizophrenic condition. This is one of the most common subtypes and is associated with a course, outcome, and prognosis which vary, depending upon the predominant type of symptoms. Significant negative and cognitive symptoms, for instance, are associated with poorer outcomes.

Residual schizophrenia is less a subtype of schizophrenia itself and more of a phase that people with the other four types of schizophrenia shift into when their condition is predominantly characterized by negative symptoms and cognitive deficits, as opposed to delusions, hallucinations, disorganization, or catatonia.

The typical course of schizophrenia is that an individual demonstrates a weeks-to-years-long prodromal phase, during which their positive symptoms are attenuated, in terms of frequency, intensity, loss of insight, and behavioral impact, and functioning gradually deteriorates (3, 4). With the transition to syndromal schizophrenia and the first-episode of psychosis, one or more positive symptoms is met with increased intensity and full loss of contact with reality. After approximately two to five years from the diagnosis of a syndromal condition, individuals leave the first-episode or early stages of psychosis and are considered to be in the chronic phase of the disorder. The first ten years of schizophrenia tend to be characterized by relapsing (often occurring in the context of severe life stressors, medication nonadherence, or substance use) and remitting symptoms. After this period, many, but not all, individuals enter the previously described residual phase.

Remy eventually entered a residual phase. Remy had been very reliably taking her medications for years and had no delusions or hallucinations of any sort. Remy had been asking her psychiatrist to stop her medication as she no longer felt that she needed it. She was very adamant about this. Unsure of what to recommend, Remy's psychiatrist was referred to the schizophrenia clinic at a New York City hospital for a consultation, where we examined her.

Remy, who was 50 years old at the time of the evaluation, looked younger than her actual age. She was approximately five feet in height, quite thin, no more than ninety-five pounds in weight, and was casually dressed in gray pants, with a light green turtleneck. She was polite and appropriate. She spoke with a slight, but noticeable, Spanish accent. She wore small amounts of makeup. She wore a crucifix around her neck. There was nothing ornate or fancy about her appearance, although she was not underdressed nor disheveled in any way. She wore small glasses and had a pale complexion. She explained to us her whole history, which was corroborated, in full, by her husband. She indicated that she would like to stop her medication because she did not feel she needed it and never thought she did. She denied any side effects.

This discussion is typical for patients suffering from schizophrenia. Even patients who are otherwise very well treated, with no side effects, often want to stop their medications. This is typically due to a lack of insight, stigma, or both. One may ask how someone with such an obvious history of psychotic symptoms may still lack insight. While we still do not know exactly why insight is so poor in schizophrenia, we do know that this is a key feature of the condition and responsible for substantial morbidity. This is one reason a robust support system, such as a family, is so important for people with the disease. Without individuals such as a family constantly encouraging people with schizophrenia to take their medications or keep appointments with doctors, it is likely that outcomes for many individuals with schizophrenia would be significantly worse.

When asked explicitly about her previous symptoms, Remy dismissed them as episodes of "stress" and explained that it is typical for people from her cultural background, especially those who are devoutly Catholic and raised in rural Valencia, to feel that they can communicate with God, hear God's voice, or feel the presence of evil spirits.

This raises an important point about cultural considerations and topics when understanding schizophrenia. Religious-themed delusions and hallucinations, such as those experienced by Remy, are remarkably common in schizophrenia, and differentiating psychotic symptoms from beliefs that may not be held by everyone, but are commonly held within certain cultures or faiths, is critical. In this case, we were able to rely on her husband, who hailed from a very similar background, to tell us that Remy's beliefs and experiences were atypical. He explained that most Catholics do not believe they can openly communicate with demons or God. This underscores the importance of collateral history when evaluating individuals with schizophrenia, especially when the delusions are not bizarre. In this case, however, even though the delusions and hallucinations were essentially implausible, there are culture-bound beliefs that might seem bizarre to some people, and not to others.

In Remy's case, for example, she believed she could communicate with God and that evil spirits were real presences, even taking command of other people to harm her and her family. Without any collateral history, cultural consultations, or other similar corroborating information by which to help guide oneself, it is critical to consider other components of a patient's history when considering whether their beliefs are more likely to be related to psychosis or to culture-bound phenomena. Several considerations to keep in mind when evaluating culture-bound phenomena versus psychosis include: 1) symptoms that are psychotic in nature are likely to be accompanied by other positive symptoms, such as delusions and hallucinations that may not be related to the same themes; 2) symptoms that are related to psychosis are often accompanied by cognitive deficits and negative symptoms, whereas thoughts or experiences related to culture-bound phenomena would be less likely related to these additional symptoms; 3) psychotic symptoms are more likely to be worse when people are not taking medications, and better or nonexistent when people are taking their medications, whereas culture-bound phenomena are less likely to respond to medications; 4) psychotic symptoms are likely to start in late adolescence or the early twenties, while culture-bound phenomena are less likely to fluctuate over the lifespan; 5) symptoms that are psychotic in nature are likely to be accompanied by functional impairment, whereas culture-bound phenomena are less likely to be related to functional impairment.

A review of Remy's symptoms and clinical course in the context of the five criteria above suggested that her symptoms were more likely related to a psychotic disorder than to culture-bound phenomena. Therefore, we discussed Remy's symptoms with her in the context of these criteria, never dismissing the importance of her faith or encouraging her to abandon it, as we wished to remain culturally sensitive. Stepping into her logic, we explained that her own faith teaches that she should not be afraid of the devil, but view him as defeated by God. She spoke of the statue from her childhood living room, showing the Virgin Mary crushing the head of the devil, and smiled. Still, however, she continued to insist that she did not need medications, that her condition was simply related to stress, and that beliefs such as hers were typical for people of her culture.

Given Remy's clear history of relapse when stopping medications, we recommended that she continue her medication. Remy indicated that she appreciated our advice and would discuss this with her psychiatrist. The next we heard about Remy was two years later. Her psychiatrist contacted us for collateral information. He filled in the recent history for us, saying that, despite our recommendations, Remy insisted on tapering her olanzapine. He agreed to help Remy taper her medication in a safe way, even though he disagreed with her plan, because he was concerned that she would simply stop the medication without a taper, which would have increased her risk of relapse and withdrawal side effects. Together, Remy and her psychiatrist tapered the medication by 2.5mg over a year, which is a very slow taper. Once Remy had tapered to 2.5mg, her symptoms returned. She began to have conversations with evil spirits, shout at them while driving, become more irritable, and talk about how she was concerned that her neighbors were in league with the devil and were coming after her. Remy's husband eventually told Remy that she had no choice but to take the full dose of her medication, which she ultimately did. Her symptoms rapidly remitted. Fortunately, this brief relapse did not result in hospitalization and Remy's medication continued to work for her. She had otherwise been functioning at her baseline, with mild negative symptoms and cognitive deficits. Although she still had mild impairment in functioning due to her negative symptoms and cognitive deficits, Remy and her family were happy and doing well. Remy's husband Juan had taken partial retirement and they were enjoying this time together. They now have four grandchildren living in Texas and California and are spending a substantial amount of time with their grandchildren.

References

1. American Psychiatric Association. *Diagnostic and statistical manual of mental disorders.* 5 ed. Washington, DC: American Psychiatric Association; 2013.
2. American Psychiatric Association. *Diagnostic and statistical manual of mental disorders.* 4 ed., rev. ed. Washington DC: American Psychiatric Association; 2000.
3. Lewis DA, Lieberman JA. Catching up on schizophrenia: natural history and neuro-biology. *Neuron.* 2000;28(2):325–334.
4. Fusar-Poli P, Borgwardt S, Bechdolf A, Addington J, Riecher-Rossler A, Schultze-Lutter F, Keshavan M, Wood S, Ruhrmann S, Seidman LJ, Valmaggia L, Cannon T, Velthorst E, De Haan L, Cornblatt B, Bonoldi I, Birchwood M, McGlashan T, Carpenter W, McGorry P, Klosterkotter J, McGuire P, Yung A. The psychosis high-risk state: a comprehensive state-of-the-art review. *JAMA Psychiatry.* 2013;70(1):107–120.

12

NEGATIVE SYMPTOMS AND COGNITIVE DEFICITS

When Petronella ("Nellie") first came to see us, she was a 20-year-old, religiously agnostic, bisexual female, born and raised in New York City until age 8. Her family then relocated to Ardsley, and then White Plains, when she was 16. She resided there with her 53-year-old father, "Donald," a retired army sergeant who worked for a local bakery. Nellie was estranged from her mother. She described her mother as having severe obsessive-compulsive disorder and alcohol abuse.

Nellie's relationship with her mother was highly conflicted, with instances of verbal and physical fights between them since the age of 15. For example, one time when Nellie was 17, they had a physical altercation, allegedly because her mother came home under the influence of alcohol and started shouting at Nellie's father, making Nellie feel they were in danger. Nellie attacked her by hitting her with a soup ladle. Nellie's mother responded by pulling her hair. The pull was so forceful that she pulled out a large clump of Nellie's hair and tore her scalp, leaving Nellie with an approximately three-inch diameter bald spot on her head. Nellie called 911 and the mother was investigated by child protective services.

When asked about other possible traumatic experiences across her lifetime, Nellie reported that, in middle and high school, she was extensively made fun of by peers, first because of her race (Nellie was mixed race), then because of the small bald spot on her head, and then because her family did not have as much money as the other people in her school. Nellie reported that she was very upset about being made fun of for these reasons, which led her to keep a chip on her shoulder.

Nellie had never been married and had no children. She reported one relationship with a 35-year-old woman whom she met online, though this relationship ended after two months. They remained friends for several years. Nellie was still interested in dating when she first came to see us, but stated that she struggled to meet new people who were interested in her. Nellie indicated that, in the future, she did want to get married and have a family, but not for a few years.

Nellie reported that she had many close friends whom she would see frequently. She would see one to two friends outside of school on a regular basis. She also enjoyed watching reality television shows and shopping at bargain clothing stores when socializing. She was also active in her school's LGBTQ center. When alone, she liked to draw circus animals.

Nellie reported that, when she was younger, she did well in school. In high school, however, her grades began to drop, which she attributed to not doing her homework. She was never held back in school and was still able to pass her classes. When we first met Nellie, she was enrolled in a community college. She was passing most of her classes, though not excelling. She reported a low drive and a sense of feeling overwhelmed with stress.

Nellie described her mood as generally low. She had a full range of affect, with occasional inappropriate smiling and laughter. No staring was noted. Her speech was normal in tone and rhythm, but occasionally loud. She described longstanding feelings of irritability, as well as sad and anxious moods, which intensified for about one to two days at a time, but never longer. She also reported anxiety attacks at times, during which she would feel somewhat "hyper" and agitated. During these attacks she would have trouble concentrating on whatever she was doing. She would also retreat from whatever she was doing. At times, these attacks were so severe that she would be unable to speak.

Nellie reported chronic thoughts that it might be better if she did not exist or if she were passively killed, since age 9. She had never had any history of actual plans or intent to commit suicide. She had cut herself on three previous occasions. She once cut herself on her wrists with a pocketknife, once used a boxcutter to cut herself on her upper thigh, and once used a cousin's katana sword to make an "X" on her lower chest. She would also occasionally chew on her fingernails until only the pulp was remaining. She indicated that she felt in control of these behaviors.

Nellie reported occasional violent thoughts toward her mother or people who reminded her of her mother, but denied any plan or intent to harm her mother. She and her father had two guns in the house, as her father was at one point an avid duck hunter, though Nellie herself had never used a gun. She had also never been arrested.

Nellie would occasionally drink alcohol with her friends. This usually occurred on weekends when she and her friends would procure beer and drink it until the point of getting drunk. She reported that she very much looked forward to becoming "wasted" with her friends. She denied that she would drive while intoxicated. She also denied that she would drink when not with her friends and otherwise denied any past or current psychosocial problems with alcohol. She rarely used marijuana as she felt that it made her "paranoid" and generally worsened her anxiety. She denied any other past or current use of illicit drugs or abuse of prescribed or over-the-counter medications.

Nellie was referred to our clinical high-risk clinic by her provider in White Plains because she was experiencing and reporting a number of unusual experiences, and that is when we first met her. She was approximately five feet, five inches tall, casually groomed in a gold-colored t-shirt and jeans. She was cooperative and pleasant, though mildly anxious. Her black hair was clean and in a ponytail. Her hair was strategically placed to cover her bald spot. Her speech had a normal prosody, rate, and rhythm. Her mood was slightly "low" and she appeared dysthymic, with a full range of affect. She also reported and/or displayed a number of positive symptoms, all attenuated in nature.

Since about age 18 or 19, Nellie felt that there may have been a fault line underneath her bedroom that became active once a night. She reported that this might have been the case because every morning when she would wake-up she would sense that the furniture in her bedroom was in a different place than when she went to sleep. She studied geological surveys of Westchester County and understood that there was no known fault line near her home, but was unable to otherwise account for her experiences. She did not find this distressing, but instead "interesting" to consider. She described this as fluctuating in frequency and intensity, relative to her stress and sad moods, and not increasing in the previous year. She also described herself as feeling guilty for the discord between her mother and father. This feeling, which occurred with high, but never complete, conviction, was vaguely associated with a sense that she might have been intensely malodorous and therefore unappealing to her parents, although there was no evidence for this. At the time, we asked Nellie if there was any significance to her feelings that she may have been responsible, or "at fault," for her parent's discord and that she thought that there may have been a fault line underneath her bedroom that was moving everything in her life on a daily basis. Nellie felt that this was an intriguing insight and hoped to be able to work on it in therapy.

Nellie was engaged and forthcoming throughout the interview, with no guardedness. She described a sense that she was disliked or alienated by her friends, intensifying over the previous year to occur nearly daily. She had been "mildly," but never completely, convinced, related to the way she perceived slight gestures, looks, and actions. She also reported concern since about the tenth grade that people on buses may have wanted to steal her phone, leading to hypervigilance when in public places in general, especially on buses. This had not been increasing in the previous year. Over the previous four years, she had sometimes felt that her extended family friends were intentionally leaving her out of family picnics and generally thought that she did not fit in with them. She reported that this happened about once a day and had been increasing in the previous year to become distressing and occur with "moderate" conviction. She denied any sense of having to prepare to arm herself or carry a weapon in the context of her suspicious ideas.

Nellie was not expansive during the evaluation process, though she would sometimes make inappropriate jokes and remarks. She was responsive to redirection in this regard. When asked about special gifts, she did endorse a longstanding, not increasing, sense of being morally superior to most other people, including family and friends, which was associated with feelings of distress when people did not appreciate these aspects of herself. She had, on occasion, refused to speak to people who did not validate these traits. In the previous year, she had thoughts, with "high," but never complete, conviction that she could do a good job as a spiritual leader to the LGBTQ community. She had endorsed occasional, vague thoughts in the previous year that, if she could somehow be appointed as a Supreme Court justice, she could do a better job of passing judgments.

Nellie did not appear internally preoccupied during the evaluation and denied perceptual disturbances in any sensory modality. She reported that she had a tendency to lose focus while speaking and talk about other things. She reported that this occurred across her lifetime, but stated that this had been happening more frequently and with more intensity in the previous year. She was somewhat circumstantial during the evaluation, sometimes requiring some redirection, to which she was responsive. Also, in the past year, she noticed that her mind would sometimes completely lose focus mid-conversation so that she would have to stop and think about what she was talking about. This occurred a few times a week. She did find it distressing. She was capable, most of the time, to regain her footing and return to her original point.

Nellie began treatment in our clinic. She received both weekly psychotherapy as well as medication management. Despite full treatment, her symptoms progressed, so that within four months she had developed syndromal schizophrenia. Over that time period, she began to think that politically conservative senators from the future were going back in time to prevent her from becoming a Supreme Court justice. She became extremely paranoid because of this delusion and began to avoid nearly any public places, including school. She continued to interact with her friends and family. She also indicated that, while she still wanted to go to public places, the risk was not worth the benefit because she had to avoid the conservative senators from the future who were looking to kill her. She also began to develop auditory hallucinations of the conservative senators from the future talking about how they were going to prevent her from sitting on the Supreme Court by killing her.

Nellie was able to make it through her transition to syndromal schizophrenia and her first-episode of psychosis with only one hospital admission, at a time when she stopped her medications because she thought that they were being replaced with poison. She continued to come to our clinic for treatment and was seen regularly in our clinic for individuals with chronic schizophrenia.

Twelve years after Nellie developed syndromal schizophrenia, her condition had changed in a remarkable manner. Nellie's delusions about being a Supreme Court justice had all but resolved. She no longer worried about conservative senators from the future trying to kill her and thereby prevent her from being appointed to the Supreme Court. She did not think that she was morally superior to other people. She had minimal residual paranoia and had almost completely abandoned her concerns about having broken up her parents' marriage due to being malodorous or for any other reason. She was no longer endorsing having a fault line underneath her bedroom. She occasionally had an auditory hallucination of her name being called, though these were infrequent and neither distressing nor distracting. When this happened, Nellie would simply not respond.

In summary, Nellie's positive symptoms had almost completely remitted. When asked about them, she would acknowledge that many of these thoughts used to be true, but reported that she no longer believed them. However, negative symptoms and cognitive deficits were now dominating Nellie's life. As described above, Nellie used to have a number of friends and would socialize on a regular basis. Nellie began spending no time with her friends and had no interest in doing so. For several years her friends would reach out to her and ask her to spend time with them. In response, Nellie would simply decline. After this happened repeatedly for several years, Nellie's friends no longer asked to spend time with her. Nellie had also given up drawing, shopping and watching television. She stated that she was no longer interested in doing these things.

Nellie would also rarely become angry, no longer had a chip on her shoulder, and was never agitated. Her anxiety had almost completely resolved. She was no longer upset about her mother and would not think about her. She did not know where her mother was and did not care to find out. Nellie would still report that she was bisexual, but was no longer interested in dating and would not pay attention to LGBTQ issues. When asked what she was interested in, she would say "nothing." She also had not had thoughts to harm herself for years. She had completely dropped out of school and stopped working. She was supported by disability payments from the federal government.

Interviewing Nellie was challenging because of how malodorous she had become. While she used to care about being malodorous as a cause for her parent's separation, Nellie now showered at most once every two weeks and when she did shower she would generally just step into the shower, get wet, and then step out. Nellie would not brush her teeth or comb her hair. Her bald spot was completely apparent and Nellie did not seem to mind. She would usually not change her clothes unless someone, usually her father, with whom she still lived, would ask her to. On interview, Nellie was cooperative and not unpleasant and would attend most of her appointments, but would not say anything unless asked. Anything she said was limited to two to three words. Her affect was almost completely flat, showing almost no reactivity to what was said or to what happened around her.

Collateral information from Nellie's father provided greater information about her life. Nellie would sleep ten to twelve hours a day. When she would wake up, she would eat very slowly, usually plain bread and cream cheese, sometimes for multiple meals a day. She would rarely prepare foods for herself. Nellie would otherwise sit around the house. The television was often on in the home since Nellie's father enjoyed watching television. Nellie would look at the screen but would not be able to say what was happening or describe the plot, the characters, or the score (if they were watching a sporting event). Nellie would occasionally leave the house when forced by her father, but otherwise would stay at home. Initially, Nellie was able to manage the bills and her disability payments, but eventually made too many mistakes, so Nellie's father had to take this over. Nellie would occasionally assist her father at the grocery store or when doing yardwork, but took no initiative of her own. She would not laugh at even the funniest jokes. Rather, when a joke was told, she would stare as if looking into space. It would be unclear if she understood the joke or if she simply found it unfunny.

What Nellie was experiencing was negative symptoms and cognitive deficits. Negative symptoms generally involve the lack of some normal function. Typical negative symptoms experienced by individuals with schizophrenia are poverty of speech and thought (alogia), decreased interest in things (anhedonia), decreased energy and motivation (anergia, amotivation), decreased affect, a general state of indifference (apathy), and decreased interest in socialization. Cognitive deficits in schizophrenia include impaired attention, worse short-term memory, and decreased higher order "executive" functions such as retaining, planning, and manipulating information. Most individuals with schizophrenia experience at least some negative symptoms and cognitive deficits, though there are a few who do not. Negative symptoms and cognitive deficits are thought to account for greater functional impairment than the positive symptoms of schizophrenia, though they are not responsive to traditional treatments, such as antipsychotic medications.

There are also "secondary" negative symptoms that may be observed as part of the side effects of antipsychotic medications. For example, some antipsychotic medications, especially older, so-called first-generation antipsychotic medications such as haloperidol and fluphenazine, lead to extrapyramidal side effects such as parkinsonism, which can include a general slowing of one's movements and blunted affect. It is also possible that depressive symptoms, such as anergia, anhedonia, and apathy, can masquerade as negative symptoms.

Because of the substantial negative symptoms that Nellie was experiencing, and because her positive symptoms had been essentially remitted for several years, Nellie and her father asked to taper her antipsychotic medications (at the time, risperidone 4mg). They were hoping that her negative symptoms would improve, at least partially. Nellie tapered her risperidone over a time period of eight months, decreasing her dose by 0.5mg every month. She experienced no worsening of her positive symptoms. However, she also experienced no improvements in her negative symptoms, even after having been off risperidone for three months. Therefore, Nellie and her father decided to remain off the risperidone. She remained stable, off medications, for many years, though remained debilitated by her negative and cognitive symptoms. While negative symptoms and cognitive deficits can be observed at any point in a person's illness, including during the clinical high-risk phase, they, by definition, dominate the residual phase of schizophrenia, as described in Chapter 11. Nellie was unambiguously in the residual phase of schizophrenia.

Therefore, we enrolled Nellie in a program of cognitive rehabilitation. While there are no approved treatments for negative symptoms and cognitive deficits, there are some therapies that, while not FDA approved, have some evidence for efficacy. For example, cognitive remediation is a type of cognitive rehabilitation that has patients repeatedly perform tasks that improve their attention, memory, planning, and other executive functions (1). These tasks are often performed on a computer and can be enjoyable, implemented in something like a video game format.

Nellie's response to cognitive remediation was mild. She attended the majority of her sessions and displayed some minor improvements in experimental tests of attention and executive functioning. Unfortunately, she demonstrated no improvements in her functioning and her improvements were otherwise not clinically relevant. Nellie's negative symptoms and cognitive deficits continued to impair her functioning. However, as Nellie's father reported at one of her most recent visits, she was not experiencing any positive symptoms. To Nellie's father, he was very happy for this reality as, while she remained very impaired, the concern that Nellie's delusions and hallucinations would return led to a chronic sense of hypervigilance and anxiety in their household. He was happy for both of their sakes that they would likely not have to worry about the very disturbing reality of having a family member in a floridly delusional and psychotic state.

While cognitive remediation was of limited benefit for Nellie, the development of these types of therapies has infused the field with hope that cognitive remediation and other similar therapies will gradually decrease the great functional burden imposed by negative symptoms and cognitive deficits experienced by people such as Nellie and allow patients and their family members of new reality where they can hope for more than a partial treatment of their schizophrenia.

Reference

1. Medalia A, Choi J. Cognitive remediation in schizophrenia. *Neuropsychol Rev.* 2009;19(3):353–364.

PART III

End-Stage (Dealing with Residual Symptoms and Treatment-Resistance)

13

CLOZAPINE AND TREATMENT-REFRACTORY ILLNESS

In the field of medicine, and especially in psychiatry, there are few true "miracles." Many first-year medical students carry the misperception that they, as physicians, will encounter a patient with a certain malady; expertly intervene, often with some treatment or procedure; watch the patient's problem resolve; and then receive adulation and self-fulfillment from having so successfully intervened in the life of another person. This is far from the truth. Most conditions are chronic and associated with long-term morbidity and mortality. Diabetes and hypertension, for instance, may respond well to medications, but cannot generally be cured. Moreover, most conditions are so environmentally determined – for example, the way diabetes and cardiovascular disease are affected by choices involving diet, smoking, and exercise – that, for the vast majority of patients and providers, dealing with them becomes a chronic struggle. Few all-out cures exist. One may think that surgeons routinely perform procedures that eliminate problems on such a level, but this is also a misperception. While some procedures can be curative and miraculous, this usually occurs only when a condition, such as a cancer, is caught very early and is causing limited morbidity.

Perhaps nowhere is this truer than in psychiatry, and especially with regards to schizophrenia. Complete cures rarely transpire. While medications can greatly help the lives of many people with the condition, schizophrenia remains a chronic problem and almost one-third will prove entirely treatment-refractory (1, 2). Negative symptoms and cognitive deficits occur in the vast majority of people with schizophrenic illness and both are extremely resistant to treatment.

It may well be that no field is more in need of miracles and cures than psychiatry. Before the period of deinstitutionalization from the 1960s through the 1980s, up to half a million people with severe mental illness were living in state psychiatric hospitals (3). Many had treatment-refractory psychotic illness, especially schizophrenia. For a number of reasons, including the advent of antipsychotic medications, many of these patients were discharged into the community with the idea that they would receive treatment at community mental health centers. Unfortunately, the latter were often underfunded. Moreover, such individuals were often too ill for general community life – and the legal system made it extremely difficult to involuntarily commit individuals with severe psychotic illness to psychiatric hospitals when their conditions intensified. The result of deinstitutionalization was that many of these people who previously required chronic hospitalization became homeless or wound up incarcerated. If ever a miracle or cure were needed, it would be for severe mental illnesses such as schizophrenia.

Gratefully, thanks to the efforts of researchers in the United States, the drug clozapine became available. Clozapine is as close to a "miracle drug" as possible for schizophrenia. It was developed in the 1960s and became available in Europe the following decade. It was quickly withdrawn from the market after numerous reports of agranulocytosis, which is characterized by an extremely low neutrophil count, and can be fatal if left untreated. The danger of the condition is that a low number of neutrophils leaves one highly susceptible to infection. There is a 1% chance of developing agranulocytosis in the first few months of treatment with clozapine. Fortunately, this risk decreases substantially after the first few months (4). Because of the potential for agranulocytosis, however, clozapine was relatively ignored until a landmark study was published in 1988 showing that clozapine is more effective than chlorpromazine, a standard antipsychotic medication, for individuals who had treatment-refractory schizophrenia (5). Since then, the FDA and other organizations have permitted the use of clozapine for treatment-refractory conditions, provided a patient's absolute neutrophil count is measured weekly for six months, biweekly for six months, and then monthly thereafter.

Clozapine is definitively superior to other antipsychotic medications for treatment-refractory conditions. It has, however, some disadvantages. Regular blood draws, as well as the risk for potentially fatal agranulocytosis, cause many individuals to refuse to take this medication. Additionally, the further side-effect burden of clozapine is substantial. More than any other antipsychotic medication, clozapine can cause marked weight gain, as well as increases in lipid levels, especially triglycerides, and abnormalities in blood glucose levels, sometimes leading to overt diabetes. Clozapine tends to be sedating and can also cause orthostatic hypotension. Clozapine also substantially decreases one's seizure threshold. Because of this, it is very important to very slowly up-titrate the dose. Clozapine can cause severe hypersalivation, or sialorrhea, especially while sleeping. It is not uncommon for people to wake up with their pillow drenched from saliva.

Clozapine can also cause myocarditis, a severe and fatal inflammation of the muscles of the heart. This usually begins with a fever and general physical complaints, and, within days, cardiac enzymes begin to rise. For this reason, it is often recommended that providers prescribing clozapine obtain routine troponin levels from patients.

Another rare, but serious and potentially deadly side effect of clozapine is gastrointestinal hypomotility. In severe cases, this can lead to ileus, or bowel obstruction and ischemia.

Importantly, clozapine has an extremely low to negligent risk of extrapyramidal side effects. In fact, neurologists sometimes use clozapine to treat individuals with tardive dyskinesia and severe motor conditions.

Despite all these potential side effects, which range from mild and common to rare and life-threatening, clozapine remains definitively superior to other antipsychotic medications for treatment-refractory conditions. Because of all these potential side effects, however, clozapine is also sorely underutilized. Many patients and families are discouraged by the potential side effects, if not downright frightened of them, or else simply do not want the burden of having their blood drawn every week. Many providers have limited experience with clozapine and/ or are too worried about litigation arising from a patient developing a severe side effect. Therefore, while clozapine is every bit a potential miracle drug for many people with schizophrenia, it is also emblematic of the challenges faced every day by patients, families, and providers.

"Anthony" is one patient for whom clozapine was truly a miracle. A lifelong New Yorker, his father's family relocated from Ireland to New York City in the early twentieth century. After passing through Ellis Island, Anthony's family lived in an apartment building near downtown, where they ran a stand that sold fruits and vegetables. Anthony's grandfather served in the US Army during World War II. Following discharge, he and the family moved into a new house on Long Island, situated in a large Irish-American, Roman Catholic community. Anthony's father found new work doing construction for a state agency where his mother was employed as a secretary. His parents met there and were married after a courtship of approximately one year. They went on to have two children, Anthony and his younger brother, "Connor."

Anthony had a typical childhood. He was an average student and enjoyed spending time with the neighborhood kids, playing baseball and soccer. In high school, he was a part of the swim team. In late adolescence, he got in trouble several times for skipping school in order to imbibe beer with his friends. He was moderately popular. He was interested in dating women, but struggled to connect with them socially due to shyness and insecurity about his appearance. After graduation, Anthony attended a local university. He majored in political science, joined a fraternity, had a large friend group, and took several trips abroad with his friends. He visited his family's homeland for the first time. Anthony became the first person in his family to graduate from college. He found a job as a teller at a bank. His affable, unassuming nature served him well and his performance at his job was regularly well-rated by his superiors.

Anthony rather abruptly developed delusions and hallucinations around the age of 23. He found himself caught up in an elaborate delusional system in which he believed that he was the rightful President of the United States and that he had been overthrown by a crime syndicate who were planning on overtaking the US government. He thought that their leader was the head of a fictional crime family who was actually a real person. Anthony would report that this mobster would speak to him and taunt him about his plans. He would report that the mobster's voice would harass and torment him, laughing at his inability to prevent the take-over or convince anyone that it was real.

Around age 24, Anthony had his first interaction with mental health services. Distraught about what he believed was happening, Anthony left work, took a train to the National Mall in Washington, DC, and began yelling at strangers about how the crime family was trying to take over the government under the leadership of the head of the family, masquerading as federal agents. He proclaimed that he was the rightful President and that only by returning him to power could his overthrow be prevented. Anthony was taken by the police to a nearby emergency room where he was admitted to a psychiatric inpatient unit and medicated. He was diagnosed with paranoid schizophrenia.

Anthony began treatment with 10mg of aripiprazole, initially responding very well. He spent five days in the hospital and had a near complete resolution of symptoms. He returned to New York and resumed his normal life, no longer pre-occupied by his peculiar and paranoid ideas or hallucinating. Within three months, however, Anthony stopped taking his medication and experienced a full relapse. This time, he was found shouting at strangers about his now resurfacing ideas in a New York City park. When he approached a police officer, he was again taken to a psychiatric hospital. The psychiatrists in the hospital initially reinitiated the 10mg of aripiprazole. This time, however, Anthony did not respond. The psychiatrists increased the dose to 20mg. Anthony was able to return home on this dose, but remained symptomatic. He attempted to go back to work, but within two days began to think that his boss and colleagues were also undercover agents and part of the syndicate against him. Anthony called his mother to tell her that he could no longer go to work. At this juncture, Anthony was not agitated or raising his voice, but had now incorporated coworkers into his delusion. Therefore, Anthony's parents took him to see the outpatient psychiatrist to whom he was referred following his first hospitalization. At first, they were unsure whether Anthony was taking his medications. An aripiprazole blood level confirmed that he was adherent. Therefore, since Anthony was no longer adequately responding to this medication, his psychiatrist prescribed risperidone. They started at 1mg twice daily and, over the course of two months, titrated up to a 6mg total daily dose. On risperidone, Anthony was calmer, but he continued to endorse his delusions and hallucinations. He still refused to go to work. Therefore, Anthony's psychiatrist switched Anthony to haloperidol, another antipsychotic medication.

Haloperidol brought minimal improvement. After several days, Anthony grew restless and irritable, with agitation and constant pacing at home. He would describe his beliefs with greater anger and upset. He began angrily speaking aloud to his hallucinations, telling the voice he was hearing that he would not allow him to take control of his government. Not knowing what to do, Anthony's parents again contacted his psychiatrist who told them to take Anthony to the nearest emergency room. There, Anthony was pacing back and forth, angrily interacting with his auditory hallucinations.

Anthony was again admitted to an inpatient psychiatric unit. He was given several rounds of lorazepam. Lorazepam did seem to deescalate him, but after four to six hours he would again become agitated. The inpatient attending physicians increased his dose of haloperidol with the assumption that Anthony was simply taking too low of a dose. They quickly achieved a dose of 10mg of haloperidol and continued to give lorazepam around the clock. Rather than improve Anthony's symptoms, however, he grew more agitated. At one point, he had to spend a few hours in a seclusion room because he began yelling at staff for standing too close to him.

We met Anthony on the unit after reviewing his chart and speaking with unit. He had slept little the previous night and was lying down in the seclusion room, intermittently talking aloud to his auditory hallucinations. He was approximately five feet, ten inches in stature. He had a youthful appearance and was slightly overweight. He had black hair which was not combed. He looked very tired and uncomfortable, like he had not slept in days. He was frowning and angry, although generally cooperative with the interview. He was wearing a wrinkled tee-shirt and denim shorts. Anthony was asked to explain what was bothering him. He described his ideas about the crime syndicate trying to overthrow the US government. He explained that they initially gained a foothold into the government by infiltrating federal agents and now had taken control of financial institutions, such as the one in which he used to work. He explained that he was being tormented by the head mobster who would laugh at him and mock him for being unable to prevent the takeover. Anthony described how uncomfortable this would make him feel and that over the past week he had been particularly uncomfortable, even to the point of feeling like he wanted to jump out of his skin. He explained that lorazepam would sometimes make him feel better, but the feeling would worsen as each day went by.

Based upon this history, akathisia – a subjective sense of restlessness – was suspected, masquerading as agitation related to worse positive symptoms. The nurses were instructed to begin propranolol, a beta blocker that crosses the blood-brain barrier, three times a day, and to decrease Anthony's dose of haloperidol by half.

At rounds the following day, the nurses explained that Anthony had responded well to these interventions. While he was still endorsing delusions and hallucinations, he was now much calmer and relaxed. He was able to sleep in his room and was much less internally preoccupied. Anthony reported that he felt minimally restless, with a better sense of control over his thoughts and the voice he had been hearing. It appeared, therefore, that Anthony was indeed experiencing akathisia and that haloperidol was also not targeting his symptoms. Consequently, the primary inpatient psychiatrists eventually discontinued this drug and began another antipsychotic medication.

The next time we heard from Anthony was approximately 15 years later. A colleague had been treating the patient in his private practice for the previous five years and had made minimal progress. The colleague requested a consultation. He was unaware that we had previously seen Anthony.

Anthony appeared for the consultation with his parents. He was now 38 years old, but appeared at least a decade older. His youthful appearance had given way to premature aging, including darkening and excess skin under his eyes, crow's feet, thinning and graying hair, and a slightly kyphotic posture. Anthony was also gaunt, having lost at least 30 pounds over the previous 15 years. Anthony and his parents updated us on what had transpired since we had last seen Anthony. After Anthony discontinued haloperidol on the unit, he initiated olanzapine, which proved moderately effective. At one point, Anthony was able to seek employment, but, on several occasions, he would accuse coworkers of being involved in his delusion and either quit or was fired. After taking olanzapine for seven years, with moderately good adherence, Anthony worked with his treaters to try several other antipsychotic medications, including ziprasidone, quetiapine, chlorpromazine, and perphenazine. In each case, he would briefly experience improvement, followed by a relapse of his symptoms. They also tried lithium, valproic acid, carbamazepine, and lamotrigine as add-on medications, with no substantial benefit. When we met with Anthony, he had not worked in several years and was rarely leaving his parents' home due to his persecutory delusions and new fears of being assassinated. Anthony now believed that the crime family had taken control of the US military and that snipers had been posted around the neighborhood, waiting for him to step out of his house to fire at him. The few times Anthony would leave his house, he would be disguised in a heavy coat, hat, and sunglasses, irrespective of the weather.

Anthony had been hospitalized several times over the previous 15 years when his symptoms were particularly intense. Each time he would spend several weeks in the hospital and be discharged following only mild improvement.

Fortunately, Anthony had not experienced many negative symptoms or cognitive deficits. Anthony's affect was intact and his cognition was minimally affected, beyond minor lapses in attention. He was generally well-groomed, appropriate, and organized. Anthony expressed desires to work and have a social life, but felt impeded by his overwhelming symptoms. Anthony had not seen any friends in years. He had been intermittently dating the same woman over the last 15 years, but would often incorporate her into his delusional system, accusing her of working against him, after which he would abruptly end the relationship. During periods of stability they would get back together. Their last break-up had been about six months prior to the consultation meeting.

Anthony and his parents did not initially recall the authors' meeting with Anthony 15 years prior, but eventually remembered the encounter. The parents were quite upset about his chronic condition. They explained that they had almost completely lost hope that Anthony's condition would improve since he had not responded well, beyond brief periods of improvement, to any antipsychotic medication. This was a tough realization for them because they had always hoped that Anthony would simply outgrow his psychotic symptoms. They were particularly unhappy that Anthony was unable to work or retain his relationship with his girlfriend whom they considered "a very nice and supportive person who didn't deserve such trouble." They were bothered that, at the age of 38, Anthony was still living with them and had accomplished little. They wanted Anthony to be independent, acutely aware of what would happen if Anthony were to try to live alone. They had tried to force Anthony to live alone on several occasions over the years and each time Anthony would stop his medications and become acutely hostile to either a neighbor or landlord. Emergency services were called several times. They could not understand how, after more than 15 years, Anthony still held on to the same delusions and hallucinations. They explained that they tried to reason with Anthony about how unlikely it was that what he was saying was true, given that nothing had happened after so much time.

We spoke with Anthony alone, following his parents' update. He explained that he was still being targeted by the crime family and that his parents simply did not understand the situation. He indicated that, while he did not yet think that his parents were directly involved in the conspiracy, he was concerned that they were being urged to give him up. He denied any desire to harm them or protect himself from them at the time and suggested that he would consider taking refuge in Mexico if the crime family were to gain influence over his parents, because at that point there would be few people left whom he could trust. Anthony would occasionally stare off into space, distracted by his auditory hallucinations. He indicated that the head mobster had recently told him that he had acquired control of the legal system. Anthony felt that it was only a matter of weeks before the US would be run by the crime syndicate and he was not sure what he could do to prevent this without being in control of the government himself. He was concerned that he would be tortured if captured.

Following a review of Anthony's history, it was clear that the next best step would be a trial of clozapine. Anthony and his parents stated that they had never previously heard of this medication. The parents were worried about the side effects, in particular agranulocytosis. Anthony refused the medication outright because of the weekly blood draws. After further discussion, during which the author reiterated the recommendation to initiate clozapine, Anthony and his parents returned home. The author spoke with Anthony's psychiatrist and shared the suggestion. He indicated that he had not prescribed it to a patient for over ten years and was not comfortable doing so. The author offered assistance with the case, including writing the prescription for the patient. The colleague reported appreciating the consultation and that he did not feel that Anthony was "the clozapine-type of patient." The author repeated the recommendation before amicably ending the discussion.

Three weeks later the author received voicemail messages from Anthony's parents and the colleague reporting that Anthony had been picked up by an ambulance after he was found at a nearby convenience store yelling at a fellow shopper to stop monitoring him in his home. He accused the shopper of working with the crime family and grabbed the shopper's bag, which he believed to contain a clandestine camera. Fortunately, Anthony, while quite agitated, had not actually assaulted the stranger. The owner of the convenience store had quickly called 911 before the situation was able to further escalate. Anthony was hospitalized later that day.

Anthony's parents and psychiatrist were distraught. They were currently trying amisulpride, which is not available in the America, because a foreign colleague had suggested that it might be worth trying. They indicated that they did not think that Anthony's condition was so severe that he would ever try to grab another person's belongings. They asked for more information about clozapine and ultimately agreed that it might be the appropriate next step. They asked for us to work with the inpatient psychiatrists as they began clozapine therapy.

Anthony was reluctant to initiate clozapine treatment, still hesitant about the blood draws. He ultimately decided to do so when the inpatient psychiatrists and his family told him that his other option would be to enter a state psychiatric hospital. Anthony began clozapine at 12.5mg at night. Over the course of four weeks he gradually achieved a dose of 350mg at night. His parents described his response as "nothing short of a miracle." By week four he was no longer experiencing hallucinations and by week six he was endorsing no delusional thinking. When asked about his previous positive symptoms, he described them as "ridiculous, childlike fantasies." He suggested that he felt that it was time for him to "grow up." He readily acknowledged that clozapine was helping him, but stopped short of accepting his diagnosis of schizophrenia, which is actually very typical for many patients who respond to antipsychotic medications. Anthony was quite social on the unit and began to look years younger. He did experience mild weight gain, substantial nighttime sialorrhea, and moderate daytime fatigue. He reported that he felt that these were acceptable side effects, given how "good" he was feeling. Anthony's parents said that they were "just happy to have their Anthony back."

We continued to see Anthony in consultation every six to twelve months for five years. He continued to take clozapine and, after one year, required only monthly blood draws. He never developed agranulocytosis. He eventually began a new job as a bank teller and began living independently. He developed a social circle again. He became engaged to the woman he had been seeing on and off. We were invited by Anthony's parents to the wedding and the shower for the couple's first child. They had sent personalized, hand-written notes, describing how none of Anthony's progress in life would have been possible without the author and that their only regret was that they had not tried clozapine earlier. We respectfully declined each invitation in the interest of maintaining appropriate boundaries between us and the patient.

Anthony's case highlights the reality and potential of clozapine. Although not every patient will respond to clozapine as well as Anthony did, many will. Year after year we encounter patients who have tried numerous medications and dealt with treatment-refractory psychosis for great lengths of time without ever having been told about clozapine or seriously considered it. In part, this is because many psychiatrists, due to a lack of experience with clozapine, do not consider the value of using it at all, or do so much later than it should have been considered. It may also be because we, as a field, do not do a good enough job of explaining the balance between therapeutic effects and side effects of clozapine to patients and their families. Whatever the reason for this, there is ample evidence that clozapine provides hope to many patients who might otherwise be relegated to the back halls of state mental institutions or to secluded areas of their own homes. Perhaps it would be optimal to aim to ensure that all patients have the opportunity to at least consider clozapine as soon as possible after meeting criteria for treatment-refractory schizophrenia – that is, after failing two full trials of anti-psychotic medications – and not only after decades of failed treatments with other medications.

References

1. Lieberman JA, Sheitman B, Chakos M, Robinson D, Schooler N, Keith S. The development of treatment resistance in patients with schizophrenia: a clinical and pathophysiologic perspective. *J Clin Psychopharmacol.* 1998;18(2 Suppl 1):20S–24S.
2. Bromet EJ, Fennig S. Epidemiology and natural history of schizophrenia. *Biol Psychiatry.* 1999;46(7):871–181.
3. Torrey EF, Entsminger K, Geller J, Stanley J, Jaffe DJ. The shortage of public beds for mentally ill persons: a report of the Treatment Advocacy Center. [cited November 3, 2019]; Available from: www.treatmentadvocacycenter.org/storage/documents/the_shortage_of_publichospital_beds.pdf.
4. Safferman A, Lieberman JA, Kane JM, Szymanski S, Kinon B. Update on the clinical efficacy and side effects of clozapine. *Schizophr Bull.* 1991;17(2):247–261.
5. Kane J, Honigfeld G, Singer J, Meltzer H. Clozapine for the treatment-resistant schizophrenic. A double-blind comparison with chlorpromazine. *Arch Gen Psychiatry.* 1988;45(9):789–796.

14

ELECTROCONVULSIVE THERAPY IN SCHIZOPHRENIA

"Norman," a 43-year-old male, was a member of a prominent upper-class German family. During World War II, his paternal grandparents had been imprisoned in a forced labor camp due to their opposition to the Nazi party. They would ultimately be liberated by allied Russian and American forces as the end of the conflict drew near. Paper manufacturers by trade, Norman's family benefited greatly from post-war reconstruction aid under the Marshall Plan. For several decades following the war, they built up a successful and profitable business in Bavaria outside of Munich. Norman's parents met in the early 1960s, quickly married, and went on to have three children over the next five years, all of whom received exceptional educations while additionally learning the value of manual labor by spending weekends and summers working in their parents' paper manufacturing plants.

Norman, who was the youngest of his siblings, was born in the early 1970s. He was delivered vaginally, at term, with no complications. All his developmental milestones were reportedly met within normal limits. Similar to his siblings, Norman benefited from fine schooling at a private gymnasium. He became fluent in German, English, and French and learned to understand Latin remarkably well. He earned top marks in nearly all his courses and was especially gifted at chemistry. Norman also excelled in sports, especially tennis and European football. The latter accomplishments were related in large part to his impressive physique. He had reached a height of six feet, three inches by the time he entered university, with a strong, athletic build.

Norman enrolled at a prestigious German university, with the desire to pursue a career in physics. He acclimated to university, both socially and academically, without difficulty. He developed several positive friendships and was even more popular than he had been in his gymnasium. He soon entered into his first romantic relationship with a woman named "Ilse" with whom he shared a mathematics course.

The subsequent three years constituted a favorable period for Norman. He continued to excel in his courses and his efforts were acknowledged by his professors who considered him unusually gifted. Norman was given the honor of working with leaders in the field at a prestigious German research institute. Additionally, in the summer before his fourth year at university, Normal had proposed marriage to Ilse, who accepted. They arranged to wed after completing school. Further, Norman was able to travel throughout Europe and the Middle East and experience diverse cultures and ways of life during his time in university. Norman's parents retired and passed their business on to their three older children, who continued their success.

In October of Norman's fourth year, shortly after German Unity Day, his behavior began to change. Metaphorically, his own internal "unity" had now begun to deteriorate. He became more irritable and impatient. He would regularly snap at Ilse and his friends and was increasingly isolative, suddenly unable to juggle and integrate the various aspects of his life. He became fully consumed by his experiments, often remaining in his laboratory until the early morning hours, sleeping a mere two or three hours and then returning to work or heading to a class. His speech became loud and pressured. Norman's friends and family found it difficult to get a word in edgewise when conversing with him and found it challenging to follow his train of thought. Norman's friends and family grew highly concerned about him, but did not know why Norman was behaving so peculiarly or how to handle the situation.

At this juncture, Norman was spending much more time with his laboratory mentor, a senior professor in physical chemistry. The researcher had also observed the changes in Norman's behavior, but dismissed these as the result of intense interest in his research and as not so atypical for people who specialize in the physical sciences. Norman's odd behavior, however, persisted and intensified. Now, in addition to irritability, sleeping less, spending markedly more time on his work and in his laboratory, and the aforementioned changes in his manner of speech, Norman began to explain to people that he was working on research that was going to "revolutionize science in a way that has not happened since the early twentieth century" and, in his mind, ultimately earn him a Nobel Prize in Physics. He began telling people that researchers from a rival laboratory at a prestigious university in Berlin were conspiring to steal his work in order to publish the findings first and take credit for his groundbreaking discoveries. This required him to take "extra precautions" both at home and at his lab. He wore sunglasses, a wide-brimmed hat, and an oversized trenchcoat anytime he went outside, irrespective of the weather. He installed three extra locks on the door to his apartment. He became more agitated and paranoid, now isolating from Ilse, and ceased all communication with his family. He withdrew from classes and spent nearly all his time working on the research he felt would revolutionize his field. Now even

Norman's laboratory mentor became concerned after observing Norman's further descent into utter distractibility, outright hostility, and markedly loud, sometimes incomprehensible, speech. Norman began to accuse his mentor of working with the team at the rival university to take credit for Norman's work. At times, the mentor would look in on Norman while he was in the lab and notice him openly conversing with himself.

One evening, Norman's parents came home to find a letter in the mail stating that they owed the equivalent of 100,000 American dollars on a credit card in their names. In the itemized list of expenditures, they found that essentially all this amount came from an online gambling website. Norman's parents were very concerned about the dramatic change in his behavior over the brief period of a few months and drove to his apartment in an attempt to intervene. There they found him pacing about, unshaven and unbathed for days, on the phone, shouting at the rival university's administrators that he would bring legal action if they did not pull their support and funding from researchers who were endeavoring to steal his intellectual property. Norman's parents confronted him about his bizarre actions, but he seemed oblivious, perseverating on the subject of the competitors secretly plotting against him.

Norman's parents eventually convinced him to visit a nearby hospital, where he was involuntarily admitted to a psychiatric unit for an episode of psychotic mania. Mania, mostly commonly observed in and associated with bipolar disorder – previously known as manic-depressive illness – is defined by the current fifth edition of the Diagnostic and Statistical Manual of Mental Disorders (DSM-5), released in 2013, as, having at least one week of elevated, expansive, or irritable mood and increased energy or goal-directed activity and at least three (or four if the mood is only irritable) of seven symptoms, including distractibility, increased involvement in activities with a high potential for danger, grandiosity, increased or pressured speech, increased psychomotor or goal-directed activity, decreased sleep, or racing thoughts (1). Norman met each of these criteria. Individuals experiencing a manic episode commonly present with positive symptoms of psychosis, such as delusions and hallucinations, and these are often paranoid and grandiose in nature, both of which we observe in the present vignette.

In the 1990s, when Norman entered the hospital, manic episodes were primarily treated with mood stabilizers, such as lithium, valproic acid, or carbamazepine. More recently, with the advent of the second-generation antipsychotic medications, most individuals experiencing manic episodes or full-blown bipolar disorder are treated with antipsychotic medications, such as olanzapine, risperidone, or aripiprazole. Norman was prescribed lithium and experienced a rapid recovery. Within two weeks, he returned to a euthymic mood state and was discharged from inpatient treatment. He displayed no psychotic symptoms, returned to school, and made amends with his family, friends, mentor, and fiancée. Norman graduated on time, married Ilse, and began working at a prestigious scientific institute in Germany.

Unfortunately, over the next few years, Norman would periodically abandon his medications, due to feeling like he no longer needed them. This would typically result in relapses resembling his first manic episode. With each relapse, however, his overall condition became incrementally worse. While he would reinitiate lithium each time with subsequent resolution of his manic symptoms, his delusions about other researchers stealing his work would persist, first for several weeks, and then, after his third relapse, for several months at a time.

The outpatient psychiatrist who was treating Norman attempted trials of valproic acid and carbamazepine, but neither did much to stem his delusional belief system. In addition, Norman's condition began to change. Rather than having very discrete episodes of severe and acute mania, he now demonstrated more mild episodes of hypomania and depression, along with inter-episode periods of delusions and hallucinatory voices, chattering away for long portions of the day. Therefore, Norman's psychiatrist prescribed antipsychotic medications, including risperidone, olanzapine, and quetiapine. Each would work for three to five years but, eventually, Norman would abandon treatment, suffer a partial relapse, and struggle to recompensate upon returning to his medications.

In his late 30s, now married with three children, Norman and his wife became increasingly concerned about his psychiatric health. He was no longer experiencing manic episodes, but rather full depressive episodes approximately once every two years. These would generally last two to three months and severely impair him. These episodes were typically characterized by markedly diminished mood and energy. His appetite was poor, resulting in significant weight loss. He would rarely participate in family activities, preferring to spend long spells in bed. He was often unable to work, which began to affect the family's finances. He would complain that he was a failed researcher – although, despite his depressive spells and lay-offs, he proved extremely productive at work – and ask God to take his life. The latter was suggestive of delusionally low self-esteem, which is often observed in the context of psychotic depressive episodes.

At this point, Norman's condition had developed into what is known as schizoaffective disorder. This condition is considered a primary psychotic disorder and is conceptualized as existing on a continuum between a major affective disorder, such as major depressive disorder or bipolar disorder, and schizophrenia. Like major affective disorders, people with schizoaffective disorder experience major episodes of depression or mania, or mixed states. Unlike people with major affective disorders, however, people with schizoaffective disorder exhibit at least two weeks of persistent psychotic symptoms, such as delusions or hallucinations, even when they do not have mood symptoms, which themselves must be present for the majority of the illness (1). (Of note, people whose symptoms meet criteria for schizophrenia may also experience major affective episodes, though they would not be present for a majority of the illness).

Schizoaffective disorder often initially appears as a major affective disorder/episode and then more clearly manifests as a psychotic illness within several months or years of the first affective episode. Appropriate treatment generally includes an antipsychotic medication with either a mood stabilizer (such as lithium) for people with predominantly manic episodes or an antipsychotic medication along with an antidepressant medication, such as fluoxetine, bupropion, or sertraline, for people with predominantly depressive episodes. It is also common for people who present with manic episodes to experience primarily depressive episodes later in the course of illness, as was the case for Norman.

By age 40, Norman had accepted the importance of taking medications and no longer had difficulties with adherence. At this point, he was taking 20mg of olanzapine and 250mg of sertraline. He and his psychiatrist had arrived at this combination after trying full courses and doses of combinations of risperidone, quetiapine, fluoxetine, and paroxetine. During one particularly severe episode, Norman presented with a delusional belief that, because of his perceived failure as a physical chemist, his children would be branded as "unintelligent" and never be permitted entry into a university. As a result, Norman felt that the only way to save his children from a lifetime of ridicule and exclusion was to take his own life. To that end, one weekend he rose early while the rest of the family was still asleep and penned a note explaining his distorted thinking. Tying a rope to a light fixture on the ceiling of his bathroom, he hanged himself. Fortunately, the fixture broke before Norman was able to permanently injure or kill himself, although he did lose consciousness. He was found by his youngest daughter who woke up after hearing the commotion in the bathroom.

Norman was subsequently hospitalized. He was now clearly suffering from a treatment-refractory form of illness, meaning that he had failed several trials of antipsychotic and antidepressant medications. He was prescribed clozapine, which is often employed in such treatment resistant cases. It is also considered to specifically possess anti-suicidal properties, as demonstrated by the seminal International Suicide Prevention Trial (InterSePT) (2).

Norman's response to clozapine was robust. Although he had to spend a full month in the hospital to allow a full dose up-titration of the drug, as well as venlafaxine, Norman experienced full resolution of his psychotic and depressive symptoms. Norman was discharged. Over the following six months, he and his family experienced a quality of life that they had not experienced in some years, although Norman's youngest daughter did experience significant emotional difficulties after finding Norman unconscious in the bathroom following his suicide attempt, for which she required psychiatric care.

Within six months of treatment with clozapine, Norman developed a cough that would not go away. He rapidly developed a severely sore throat, high fevers, and rigors. He went to an emergency room and was found to have 100 neutrophils per mm^3 of blood. Norman had developed agranulocytosis. This condition most commonly develops in the first few months of clozapine use and is very rare, though not impossible, thereafter. The only treatment was to immediately stop clozapine, which Norman did. His neutrophils recovered, as did his medical condition. Given his severe reaction to clozapine, however, he was not able to reinitiate clozapine. He instead returned to olanzapine and venlafaxine and experienced substantial, though not complete, resolution of his psychiatric symptoms.

A few months later, Norman came to New York City for an academic meeting for international researchers. On the second morning of the conference, Norman was found by bystanders in a parking lot with self-imposed, deep lacerations to both of his wrists. He was bleeding to death. Emergency services were called and Norman was taken to the hospital where he received medical treatment. After he was medically stabilized, Norman was admitted to a Manhattan hospital, where we first encountered him.

We met Norman on one of the facility's inpatient units. He was tall and extremely thin, almost gaunt in appearance. He was pleasant, cooperative, and courteous, speaking fluent English with a subtle German accent and minimal intonation to his voice. He was overtly depressed, but never tearful. His affect was blunted and rarely changed, with no smiling or frowning at any point. He spent most of his time on the unit isolating to this room, although he did no reading there. His speech was organized and coherent. He displayed limited insight and impulse control. Norman explained to us his beliefs that he was a failure as a scientist, would never win the Nobel Prize, and that, because of his shortcomings, his children would be blacklisted from academia. He explained that he had to kill himself in order to give his children the opportunities that they deserved. Norman explained that he loved his family, which was unmistakable, and that he was sorry for his own existence, for their sakes.

We placed Norman on constant observation in light of his risk for self-harm and considered Norman's options. Clozapine would have been ideal for Norman given his suicidality and prior response, but it was considered too risky due to previous agranulocytosis. We discussed these ideas with Norman and recommended that he try electroconvulsive therapy (ECT), which is known colloquially as "shock treatment." This intervention employs electricity to induce a seizure and is one of the most effective treatments in all of medicine. It is primarily used for treatment-resistant major affective disorders, such as major depressive disorder and bipolar disorder, and may be effective for schizoaffective disorder or schizophrenia, especially when they include significant mood components, as was the case for Norman, or substantial catatonia. The induction of seizures for psychiatric treatment has been used in psychiatry for decades. Before ECT, people would sometimes use camphor oil or high-dose insulin to induce seizures. These practices are extremely dangerous. ECT became more popular and widespread in the early to mid-twentieth century, even before the development of modern psychopharmacology, which refers to medication treatment in psychiatry.

There is considerable stigma surrounding the use of ECT, primarily due to portrayals in the media, such as in some popular movies. The mechanism of action of ECT is currently unknown, but it is considered a very safe procedure with which the field has great experience. During ECT, which is typically performed in the presence of an anesthesiologist, patients are given general anesthesia and then a muscle relaxant to induce paralysis. An electrical current is then administered to one of their temples – usually the right; bitemporal ECT is used on occasion, as bitemporal ECT is somewhat more efficacious, but also associated with more substantial amnesia. This produces a brief seizure, usually lasting approximately 60 seconds. Patients are unconscious and their muscles relaxed during the seizure, so they do not experience anything themselves. Following the procedure, patients recover quickly. In many cases, patients resume normal activities within one hour. People with affective conditions infrequently require more than eight to 12 sessions of ECT, while it is not uncommon for individuals with psychotic disorders to require more than 12 in order to achieve remission.

Norman consented to and initiated ECT. He experienced little benefit after his first few administrations, but did begin to experience substantial lifting of his mood following his sixth to eighth treatments. He continued to experience gradual but definite improvements in his mood and psychotic symptoms through his 14th and 15th sessions, at which point we reinitiated olanzapine and venlafaxine. After two months in the hospital, Norman experienced a complete remission of his psychotic and depressive symptoms. He no longer felt suicidal, felt "happy," and denied any delusions. When we would ask him about his previous belief systems, he acknowledged that he had become caught up in these ideas in the past and that they felt somewhat plausible, but that he did not feel the same about them now. He was able to see himself as a successful individual. Norman was eager to return to Germany, see his children, and get back to work. His wife had traveled to New York several times during Norman's hospital stay. Norman was discharged from the hospital after ten weeks on the unit. He continued maintenance ECT sessions every six to eight weeks, as well as olanzapine and venlafaxine for at least three years post-discharge. He experienced mild changes in his mood over that time period, but no longer experienced major affective episodes, delusions, or desires to end his life. He continued his success at work and made it a point to check in with us every six months to a year, or when he was in New York, saying he was doing well and had been able to keep himself out of the hospital.

Norman's case, while severe in nature, is, in some respects, typical of treatment-refractory psychotic affective conditions. One very important concept it demonstrates is that of tachyphylaxis. This term refers to a diminished response a patient might experience to the same or higher doses of a medication (3). This is quite common among medications that work on the central nervous system. Additionally, this tends to be most apparent in the treatment of psychotic disorders after a person stops a medication and relapses. Afterward, such patients would typically restart a medication that had previously been efficacious, even only a few days or weeks before, and experience less of a response or none at all (4). Furthermore, the number of psychotic episodes or relapses themselves seems to enhance this effect. In addition to suggesting a "limited neurodegeneration" in psychotic disorders, these phenomena contribute to treatment-resistance and highlight the importance of maintaining adherence with one's prescribed anti-psychotic medication regimen. Treatment-resistance in schizophrenia and related disorders is quite severe and constitutes a "worst-case scenario." Fortunately, however, there are treatments, such as clozapine and ECT, which help some patients. Unfortunately, neither ECT nor clozapine is effective for all people whose symptoms are treatment-refractory. Thus, these conditions reinforce the importance of both early and sustained intervention in schizophrenia and other psychotic conditions.

References

1. American Psychiatric Association. *Diagnostic and statistical manual of mental disorders*. 5 ed. Washington, DC: American Psychiatric Association; 2013.
2. Meltzer HY, Alphs L, Green AI, Altamura AC, Anand R, Bertoldi A, Bourgeois M, Chouinard G, Islam MZ, Kane J, Krishnan R, Lindenmayer JP, Potkin S. Clozapine treatment for suicidality in schizophrenia: International Suicide Prevention Trial (InterSePT). *Arch Gen Psychiatry*. 2003;60(1):82–91.
3. Li M. Antipsychotic-induced sensitization and tolerance: behavioral characteristics, developmental impacts, and neurobiological mechanisms. *J Psychopharmacol*. 2016;30(8):749–770.
4. Lieberman JA, Sheitman BB, Kinon BJ. Neurochemical sensitization in the patho-physiology of schizophrenia: deficits and dysfunction in neuronal regulation and plasticity. *Neuropsychopharmacology*. 1997;17(4):205–229.

15

MEDICAL CONDITIONS THAT CAN MASQUERADE AS SCHIZOPHRENIA

In this chapter, we will present the story of "George," our final clinical vignette. We will also review the latest research being conducted at the New York State Psychiatric Institute/Columbia University Irving Medical Center and in the field in general through the story of George. George had persistent and refractory auditory hallucinations that proved resistant to every medication he had ever tried, including clozapine. He had thus learned to live with the voices that constantly plagued him. He was eventually referred to the New York State Psychiatric Institute to participate in a research clinic where, during the course of routine eligibility screening, a discovery was made that changed the course of his illness and life.

George was a 44-year-old heterosexual Reformed Jewish Caucasian male who was referred to a schizophrenia clinic by his private psychiatrist in rural upstate New York in the context of refractory hallucinations. At the time of intake, he resided in a house with his wife and three children. He had worked in a public library system since he graduated from high school, more than 25 years before his presentation. He reported positive relationships with his wife of 20 years, who worked as a bank teller, and their three children, the eldest of which had just begun college, and the younger two of which were attending high school.

George described himself as "always half decent" socially, denying any decline in social functioning over time. He described four meaningful friendships with people he would see at least once or twice a month. He was occasionally somewhat shy around strangers, with some wariness at times, but, as per George, never outside of the "normal range." He reported that, before he met his wife, he had one meaningful romantic relationship which lasted several months and ended because "it just didn't work out."

George met his wife, "Rachel," when he was 21. The bank at which Rachel worked was very near to the library at which George worked. They were both on their lunch break when George noticed Rachel sitting alone at a table, eating a sandwich. He approached her and they developed a very strong, long-lasting relationship.

Beyond being assessed for a learning disability in childhood, George denied any history of seeing a mental health professional prior to age 23, when he began seeing his psychiatrist in rural upstate New York, who provided medication management for his symptoms, as described below.

George's psychiatrist referred him to the research clinic due to "completely treatment refractory schizophrenia." As per his self-report, around the age of 23, George began to hear sounds that other people were not able to hear. In particular, he first would hear a constant "whooshing" sound that migrated from seeming to be in or near his head to later feeling external to his head. He experienced these sounds as clearly coming from far away, such as if one were parked at a beach and could hear waves forming and crashing.

George reported that, within a year or two of the first appearance of the sounds, he began to hear muffled voices, and then louder voices, which sometimes shouted things at him like "Hey!" or "Dumb!" He never heard more than one word at a time. He would often hear the voices along with "a sound like an air conditioner" in the background. The hallucinations tended to be worse and more frequent in the morning. George reported that, at first, the voices and sounds were very bothersome and he actively sought out treatment. Within the first several years of his hallucinations he tried a long string of psychiatric medications, including aripiprazole, ziprasidone, quetiapine, olanzapine, haloperidol, chlorpromazine, perphenazine, and risperidone. He also had trials of a number of antidepressants, lithium, valproic acid, carbamazepine, and lamotrigine. He experienced a very mild effect with olanzapine, which he took for several years. Through the early years of his condition, George continued to function well at home and at the library.

After several years of taking olanzapine, George spoke with his psychiatrist about further options for treating his hallucinations. After some deliberation and consideration of potential side effects they decided to try clozapine and eventually titrated up to a full dose of 350mg. He took it for a year with little benefit, gaining ten pounds and developing significant sialorrhea. Therefore, George cross-titrated back onto olanzapine, on which he remained for over 15 years, coming to accept the refractory nature of his hallucinations.

George visited the research clinic after reading online about the studies conducted there. As he was approaching retirement age, he thought it might also be a good time to learn more about his condition and contribute, in some way, to science, helping other people with symptoms like his. At intake, George was found to be approximately five feet, ten inches tall, casually dressed in jeans and a t-shirt. He was pleasant, calm, and taciturn. His described his mood as "good," with full affect. No significant behavioral disorganization was noted. He denied delusions or abnormalities of thought content, and none were in evidence, although he reported some uncertainty at times about whether other people could hear the same things he was hearing, prompting him to sometimes look around to see if anyone else seemed to be responding. He reported that he had previously been told he had schizophrenia.

Based on George's history and mental status examination, we were not sure about the diagnosis of schizophrenia. Therefore, with George's consent, we obtained collateral information from the patient's wife and psychiatrist, who provided the aforementioned history. The psychiatrist explained that he had interpreted George's tendency to speak so little as a negative symptom. George's wife reported that George had always been a "quiet" person, with no noteworthy change in his degree of talkativeness over the years.

As it did not appear that George's symptoms were best accounted for by a diagnosis of schizophrenia, we enrolled him in a study involving people meeting criteria for DSM psychotic disorders other than schizophrenia. This involved a Magnetic Resonance Imaging (MRI) scan and some questionnaires.

MRI uses magnetic waves to take pictures of an individual's brain. It is a critical tool used by psychiatric researchers. In contrast to computed tomography (CT) scans, sometimes called CAT scans, which primarily examine bone and blood, the MRI method is especially good for imaging soft tissues, such as the brain itself. The process has yielded some key findings in the area of schizophrenia, such as that individuals with the disorder tend to have larger lateral ventricles (the fluid-filled spaces in the brain) and small overall brain volumes than unaffected people (1). Individuals with schizophrenia also have smaller hippocampi, located in the brain's medial temporal lobe area. A number of researchers have also reported abnormalities in the so-called "white matter" of the deeper parts of the brain, containing nerve fibers, called axons, which are extensions of neurons.

Functional MRI (fMRI) uses MRI to assess the function, rather than just the structure, of the brain, either at rest or when performing certain tasks. Studies employing this technique have shown that individuals with schizophrenia have decreased function of the prefrontal areas of the brain, which are involved in complex cognitive functions. The latter include executive functioning, planning, decision-making, and socializing.

MRI is also able to measure the chemicals known as neurotransmitters in the brain. These transmit signals across chemical synapses between nerve fibers. In particular, a method known as Magnetic Resonance Spectroscopy (MRS) is able to measure glutamate, the most abundant excitatory neurotransmitter in the brain. People with schizophrenia tend to have elevated levels of glutamate in their hippocampi and prefrontal cortices when compared with unaffected individuals (2, 3).

Brain chemicals can also be measured using the nuclear medicine technologies known as Positron Emission Tomography (PET) and Single-Photon Emission

Computed Tomography (SPECT). Used primarily by physicians to examine whether a cancer has spread, PET and SPECT have revealed that individuals with schizophrenia have increased transmission of the neurotransmitter dopamine in the striatum (4–10). It is thought that excess dopamine transmission might be related to the positive symptoms of schizophrenia. Similar research has suggested that decreased dopamine transmission in frontal regions of the brain may be related to the negative symptoms seen in the disease.

Genes are also important in schizophrenia. Abnormalities in a number of genes have been found to play some role in the condition (11). Recent and very interesting research has implicated complement genes associated with the immune system (12, 13). Aberrations in some of these genes have been shown to be related to some brain abnormalities observed in individuals with schizophrenia.

Currently there are many lines of research in the area of schizophrenia, with numerous efforts to develop and test new and experimental medications. The antipsychotic medications presently available are useful, particularly for posi-tive symptoms, but, unfortunately, none is without its shortcomings. For example, there are still a substantial number of patients with schizophrenia whose positive symptoms do not respond at all to such medications, or else respond only partially. In addition, they carry many side effects, such as weight gain and, especially among the older agents, tardive dyskinesia. In addition, our current mediations have very limited to no benefit for negative symptoms or cognitive deficits. The field, there-fore, is expending considerable effort, time, and resources to develop medications with fewer side effects and that might address negative symptoms and deficits in cognitive abilities.

In short, in order to develop new treatments, we must first endeavor to more fully understand the biology and causes of schizophrenia. To these ends, many researchers are using MRI, MRS, PET, genetics, and other technologies to better explore the brain and the condition.

There is also a lot of work involving early intervention in schizophrenia. As previously noted, the earlier a patient with schizophrenia receives treatment, the better the long-term outcome. Therefore, much research is exploring how to identify schizophrenia as early as possible, including how to identify who among individuals deemed to be at clinical high-risk (CHR) for psychotic illness will ultimately develop full-blown schizophrenia. Many investigators are seeking how to best ensure that individuals in the early stages of schizophrenia receive optimal clinical care, with as few as possible falling out of treatment.

George enrolled in an MRI study and participated in a scan. The next day, we received the radiologist's report and were shocked to find that George's brain actually looked very normal, except that he had a small tumor in his auditory cortex, part of the temporal lobe region of the brain responsible for processing sounds. It was unclear, though very possible, that this tumor was responsible for his hallucinations. As George had never had a brain scan before, it was unclear how long the tumor had been present.

We spoke with George about the MRI finding. He was quite interested to hear about the tumor, asking if it was responsible for his hallucinations. We explained that this was possible, but that we could not be sure. George was given a referral to a neurologist and a neurosurgeon, whose messages to the patient were consistent with ours. They said it was certainly possible that the tumor was chronic and responsible for George's hallucinations, but they could not be certain. George inquired how dangerous the tumor was and about whether it could or should be removed. The neurologist and neurosurgeon informed George that, based on everything they knew about the tumor, it seemed like a benign meningioma. They recommended that George receive repeat MRI scans every three months for a year and then consider his options. They also recommended that George take an antiepileptic (e.g., anti-seizure) medication, but he demurred.

We saw George approximately one year later when he stopped by our offices after an appointment with his neurosurgeon. George reported that he was retired and enjoying his life, but that hallucinations were the only problem with his life. He also reported that he had been trying to lose weight and was concerned about his health, but found it difficult given that he was on medications. George indicated that the neurosurgeon told him that his tumor had not changed in size at all over the previous year and that the safest thing to do was to leave it be as it had likely been present for over 20 years. George, however, wanted to experience life without the hallucinations. He told his neurosurgeon that he understood the risks of a surgery and also understood that it was possible that the tumor was not responsible for his hallucinations, but wanted the chance to live his life without hallucinations that he opted for an elective surgery. He reported that part of the reason that he made this decision was that he had already retired and felt that it was the right time for a brain surgery, as he "had all the time in the world" and was "only going to get older."

The next and final time we saw George was two years later. The surgery had proved a complete success, with no complications and, miraculously, George's hallucinations completely resolved immediately afterward. George took anti-seizure medications for a year after his surgery, stopping about a year before this final inter-action. He was also no longer taking antipsychotic medication and had lost ten pounds. George had stopped by to express his gratitude for having come across the research program, which he felt had led to his referrals to the neurologist and neuro-surgeon and, ultimately, the resolution of his chronic hallucinations. The research team found itself hoping that, one day, new treatments would make it possible for everyone with psychotic symptoms to recover as completely as George had.

References

1.   Keshavan MS, Tandon R, Boutros NN, Nasrallah HA. Schizophrenia, "just the facts": what we know in 2008 Part 3: neurobiology. *Schizophr Res.* 2008;106(2–3):89–107.

2. Poels EM, Kegeles LS, Kantrowitz JT, Javitt DC, Lieberman JA, Abi-Dargham A, Girgis RR. Glutamatergic abnormalities in schizophrenia: a review of proton MRS findings. *Schizophr Res.* 2014;152(2–3):325–332.
3. Kraguljac NV, White DM, Reid MA, Lahti AC. Increased hippocampal glutamate and volumetric deficits in unmedicated patients with schizophrenia. *JAMA Psychiatry.* 2013;70(12):1294–1302.
4. Carlsson A. The current status of the dopamine hypothesis of schizophrenia. *Neuropsychopharmacology.* 1988;1(3):179–186.
5. Davis KL, Kahn RS, Ko G, Davidson M. Dopamine in schizophrenia: a review and reconceptualization. *Am J Psychiatry.* 1991;148(11):1474–1486.
6. Lieberman JA, Sheitman BB, Kinon BJ. Neurochemical sensitization in the pathophysiology of schizophrenia: deficits and dysfunction in neuronal regulation and plasticity. *Neuropsychopharmacology.* 1997;17(4):205–229.
7. Laruelle M, Abi-Dargham A. Dopamine as the wind of the psychotic fire: new evidence from brain imaging studies. *J Psychopharmacol.* 1999;13(4):358–371.
8. Kapur S. Psychosis as a state of aberrant salience: a framework linking biology, phenomenology, and pharmacology in schizophrenia. *Am J Psychiatry.* 2003;160(1):13–23.
9. Howes OD, Kapur S. The dopamine hypothesis of schizophrenia: version III – the final common pathway. *Schizophr Bull.* 2009;35(3):549–562.
10. Pycock CJ, Kerwin RW, Carter CJ. Effect of lesion of cortical dopamine terminals on subcortical dopamine receptors in rats. *Nature.* 1980;286(5768):74–76.
11. Harrison PJ, Weinberger DR. Schizophrenia genes, gene expression, and neuropathology: on the matter of their convergence. *Mol Psychiatry.* 2005;10(1):40–68; image 5.
12. Sekar A, Bialas AR, de Rivera H, Davis A, Hammond TR, Kamitaki N, Tooley K, Presumey J, Baum M, Van Doren V, Genovese G, Rose SA, Handsaker RE, Schizophrenia Working Group of the Psychiatric Genomics Consortium, Daly MJ, Carroll MC, Stevens B, McCarroll SA. Schizophrenia risk from complex variation of complement component 4. *Nature.* 2016;530(7589):177–183.
13. Schafer DP, Lehrman EK, Kautzman AG, Koyama R, Mardinly AR, Yamasaki R, Ransohoff RM, Greenberg ME, Barres BA, Stevens B. Microglia sculpt postnatal neural circuits in an activity and complement-dependent manner. *Neuron.* 2012;74(4):691–705.

CONCLUSION

Schizophrenia is the quintessential psychiatric disorder. It is common, disabling, and terrible. Millions of people in the USA alone struggle with this severe condition. Many of these individuals do not struggle alone. Their family and friends join in their struggle. Like no other conditions, psychiatric conditions, especially conditions such as schizophrenia, can affect the whole family. Schizophrenia is also one of the most, if not *the* most, stigmatized condition in all of medicine. The public view of schizophrenia is often that it is morality-based and primarily associated with substance use and mass violence, in many cases a result of images of the homeless, media depictions of psychotic killers, and the entertainment industry's exploitation of mental illness for dramatic purposes. The professional view is one of intractable symptoms and inexorable mental deterioration due to miseducation.

It is for these reasons that we wrote this book – to educate clinicians and the interested lay public about psychosis and many of the important clinical aspects of psychosis in both an educational and engaging way. While the prognosis for someone with schizophrenia in the early twentieth century was grave, physicians and the public alike should now feel optimistic when dealing with someone with schizophrenia. The development of antipsychotic medications in the mid twentieth century, the development of clozapine and other antipsychotic medications in the later twentieth century, and the understanding of the importance of early intervention have revolutionized what it means to have schizophrenia. Most afflicted individuals are responsive to treatment and are able to live independent, happy, and productive lives. For the minority of individuals with treatment-refractory illness, there is hope that current or soon-to-be-developed treatments will improve upon their condition. We wish to leave the reader with the further hope that, like many of the great scourges of humankind, such as polio, cancer, and smallpox, we will overcome schizophrenia on both personal and worldwide scales. This journey starts with being informed and educated about what schizophrenia is. We hope that this book has contributed to this objective in some small way.

INDEX